The food anthropologist

... a one year journey through food challenges

H. Sofia de Campos Pereira

To my homies, Patrick, Sara and Tomas, who let me fly while staying anchored.

CONTENTS

ACKNOWLEDGMENTS

Oh my! I get emotional just thinking about all of you that supported me and encouraged me throughout this project. I want to start by mentioning my clients, who trust me and constantly inspire me to want to learn more. Thanks to you, I sought to go further in my food journey, and am likely going to be a better health coach because of this experience. I am also grateful to all my family and friends who put up with me this year. To those that stayed engaged through my consecutive limitations and experiments, personally or on social media, thank you so much for your input, encouragement, and humor. Thank you for your patience as well, especially if you had the misfortune of sitting at a table and shared a meal with me when I ate only a portion of what was being served, or worse yet, didn't eat at all. Not only was your support essential, but your questions, thoughts, criticisms, and doubts were also precious, undoubtedly helping me to finalize a more interesting product. I must also thank my teachers throughout the times, who gently pushed me to always go slightly beyond my current comfort zone in any project I decided to take on. These include Marla Sokolowski (my PhD supervisor), Wanda Viegas (my boss at the University in Lisbon) and Joshua Rosenthal (founder and professor at the Institute for Integrative Nutrition). You all inspired and encouraged me to become who I am, and I could have never done this without you. My health coach, Patricia Oliveira, also deserves special mention. For being patient with me when I was losing it during tough times in some of the challenges, for encouraging me when I was feeling weak, for brain storming when I needed it and supporting me throughout with great recipes. For that, together with our great walks by the sea every other Friday, thanks! To my closer circle of friends and family, a warm thanks for all your support as well as for your concern over what these challenges may be doing for my health. Mom, I am fine, ever after eating a load of fat for a month! Lastly, and most importantly, I thank my husband and kids, who live with me and put up with me daily. Patrick, Sara and Tomas, I could not have done this without you! As much as I tried not to interfere in your eating choices, I know it did and I thank you for being flexible and taking it in stride. I am also extremely grateful for your constant support, love, and for bearing with to my endless discussions of food and food theory. I love you and thank you and can only strive to be my best self because of you.

INTRODUCTION

"And here we are at the beginning, even though it is the end that we tend to focus on and the process itself that counts."

I can't believe that my thirty-day food challenges project, including this book, has finally reached a point that I consider it to be sufficiently ready to make public. It has been a very interesting year, and I am happy to be able to share it with you. Not only was the experience of doing twelve consecutive challenges quite the trip, completing the book itself brought on a whole new set of interesting obstacles. Even now, I cannot read what I wrote without fixing it… and this is probably the fifth or sixth time I edit this particular piece of text. Objectivity is particularly difficult. It helps that I love to read and to write, and have written a lot in my life, starting with a diary as a kid and evolving to small articles, manuscripts for science journals, scientific projects, website text, blogs, newsletters, and so on… but a book… a self-edited and self-published book?! This is huge!

Digging into my mental archives, I realize that the concept of writing a novel has crossed my mind many times throughout the years. Decades ago as an adolescent I wanted to write romantic fiction, and would often invent long drawn out stories with dramatic characters and complex plots. In the end, the story lines always seemed too cheesy to me to be worth the dedication, returning the idea of publishing a book into a dream for another time. More recently, I again thought of the possibility of a novel, and believe a fantastic bestseller could have evolved from the amazing plethora of head scratching personal and family situations that I have experienced over the last decade. But that would be too personal, and I don't feel comfortable with the idea of going into other people's intimate lives in a public forum. Funny that in the end, my first book turned out to be about intimate behaviors, but they are my intimacies.

If we consider that food is the prime material used to construct our physical selves, eating is likely the most intimate thing that we do in our lives. Not only does the food we eat make up our bodies and brains, eating is likely the only thing besides sleeping and going to the bathroom that we do daily and many times a day from the day we are born to the day we die. In that sense, this is a book about my intimate food behaviors. It was precisely the food challenges that motivated me to write down my experiences, thoughts, plans, and even brain farts, and those entries that eventually allowed for the construction of this work. Truth be said, the final product required a load of dedication, time, and the staying power to reach that point where I can let it go, stop "fixing it", and to pass it on. If you are now reading it, then it somehow became possible, and I am happy and proud to present to you the final product. I hope you enjoy it.

Many years back in first-year psychology class at university, I remember learning that beginnings and endings leave a bigger mark on us than what is in between them. Personally, I do believe that beginnings set the tone, and that first impressions are important. Maybe due to the relevant role of this particular beginning, and worrying as to how it will influence your opinion of the entire work, I don't really know how best to start. What I would really like is for you to have a positive experience throughout the entire book, from the beginning to the end. If you find that some of the content gets too much into scientific details for your liking, I apologize and strongly suggest you just skip those sections. I have tried to write in such a way that it is always worth continuing to read, even after having skipped a part that you didn't particularly enjoy. But back to the beginning. I will start by introducing myself so you can get a better hang of who I am, and then we can let things evolve from there. The last thing I want is for you to be bored already, so if you are not interested in me, you can skip the next four or five paragraphs completely.

As I just mentioned earlier, I will first introduce myself and then we will let things go from there. The reason I say this is because although this book is about me and my twelve month-long food projects, I am hoping that as you read through my daily logs and divagations, it will become more and more about you and your own personal journey and self-exploration. But now, here goes me. My name is Sofia, I am an almost fifty-two-year-old Portuguese woman. I was born and lived in Lisbon Portugal for the first decade of life and then moved to Canada (mostly Toronto) a few years after the revolution in Portugal in 1974. In the mid-nineties and after living twenty years in Canada, I moved back to Portugal with my Dutch husband Patrick, who I met in graduate school in Toronto and to whom I am married to since 1993. We got married so he didn't have to go back to Holland when his student visa expired after finishing his masters in organic chemistry. I never thought I would be into a long-term relationship, but serendipity was on my side at that decision point.

Except for a couple of years in San Francisco in 1999 and 2000, we have been living close to Lisbon in a beautiful small town on the ocean fifteen kilometers west of Lisbon for more than two decades. Also, the math says that I am married for almost twenty-four years to Patrick and living together for more than a quarter of a century. Luckily for me, he is an amazing man who is my partner, best friend, lover, beach ultimate team mate, techie, and whatever else I need him to be. I hope to be the same for him. We also have two kids, Sara and Tomas, who are right now highly interesting teenagers and who we both adore infinitely. No, things are not always perfect, and there are some tough moments and phases. But overall, my immediate family of four provides me with an enriching and loving home environment where we all allow each other to fly while feeling unconditional love.

Although my immediate nucleus of four were most present for this food journey, this does not take away merit from all the other family members and friends that are a part of my life and make me who I am. Our social life is reasonably rich, with a wide circle of friends such as work and school friends, friends from disc and family friends, living on many corners of the globe as well as close by. We also live within a few kilometers of many members of my family, who I collectively and individually care about immensely, and even if I am not necessarily involved in their daily lives, learn continuously from. My mom is the third daughter of a large and close family, so there are frequently family celebrations. I could write extensively about the complex and wonderful relationships with my parents, brothers, step-mom, ex step-dad and sibs, cousins, friends and so on and so forth. However, this is not a book about my personal relationships, it is a book about food experiments.

As far as my education, I have a hard-core science background. When I started university in Toronto Canada, I wanted to be a doctor. After a few years as a biology and chemistry undergraduate student, I fell in love with research and fundamental science during first and second year summer jobs getting paid to do research in the laboratories of the biology department. In 1995, I completed a PhD at York University in Toronto, which was focused on behavior genetics of complex feeding behavior and had a strong component of molecular and neuro-biology. After that, I moved to Lisbon and spent two decades as a post-doc or research fellow doing research, orienting students, teaching, and basically focusing on fundamental science. My first post-doctorate was at the Faculty of medicine in Lisbon University studying early embryonic development. Since the early 2000s, I have been doing research at the Instituto Superior de Agronomia where my interests widened to include functional genetics of crop plants. I am still involved in research and continue to dedicate some of my time to projects, meetings and hard-core science publications, but my full-time job since January 2016 is as a health coach.

There are many reasons why my life changed from that of being a full-time scientist and researcher to that of being a health coach who also does science. For one thing, due to current economics and world politics, or perhaps increasing awareness of these issues as my years advance, my passion for fundamental science was slowly surpassed by the desire to make a more practical difference in the world. Luckily and at a friend's suggestion while in Abu Dhabi in the spring of 2015, I embarked on a one year health coach training program at the Institute for Integrative Nutrition in New York. I loved the course. It provided an ideal integrated approach to health, a comprehensive and highly practical coaching curriculum, and plenty of intelligence and additional resources to inspire me to study further. To sum up this part quickly, I will conclude that I have no doubt that being a health coach is what I am meant to do right now. I take a very scientific approach to coaching my clients, and believe that knowledge is power when it comes to our biology. Such a complex issue. I am a strong advocate of the complete integration between our body and mind, they are in truth one whole. Which, by the way, is the origin of the word health, whole. Needless to say, the whole of health is my passion right now. If you want to know more about my education or what I do, feel free to check out my website (www.besthealth.life) or Facebook page (https://www.facebook.com/besthealthbestlife/).

There is one more thing that I must mention very quickly to sum up this part "all about me". I am highly interested in athletic performance and sports, and the concept of sustainably pushing our bodies beyond their current limits. Although I am personally not a sports expert, I have close friends that I consider sports gurus who are critical in my learning process and provide me with great discussion and criticism. Also, I provide consulting in nutrition and coaching to Ultimate frisbee athletes through the Ultimate Athlete Project and, as you will read later, started following their comprehensive training plans. Personally, I love to push my body to its limits and beyond, and still practice beach ultimate regularly, which is a dynamic team sport played rectangular field with dimensions of twenty-five meters width and seventy-five meters length on sand. To feel good, I need to move, to push until I am exhausted, and to stretch. Flexibility, endurance and strength are key for a good life, and I need and work on all three regularly.

Considering that the formalities are out of the way, we can start to get into the fun stuff, the work at hand. Bear with me, I know that up to now this is a bit too much about me… hopefully that will change as you read and get inspired to explore. I really hope that you can connect with some of the things you read and turn them into part of your reality. It's all about making connections, getting inspired, and then creating your own path. In the perfect world, you will think about what you read and apply it or use it in a positive way in your life. Let me tell you how this work was born. At this point I am not sure what the final title of this book will be, but the manuscript is saved in my computer with the name "the food anthropologist". And that is the best way to describe it; a one year long journey and exploration through twelve food regimes which are currently followed by many around the world. Initially inspired by my desire to help a client that wanted to try to take gluten out of her diet, this adventure turned out to be a twelve month stint of consecutive thirty-day challenges involving various food (and beverage) limitations.

The experimental period was from May 2016 to May 2017, and the time length of each of the twelve experiments was always twenty-nine or thirty days. Since I decided to use the day of the month rather than to actually count out thirty days for each challenge, the first nine experiments started on the fifth of each month and ended on the third of the following month, with the fourth being a much looked forward to day off where there were no food limits. The tenth challenge, the paleolithic diet, happened to be in February, which only had twenty-eight days in 2017. To ensure consistency, this challenge was therefore prolonged until the fifth of March and therefore shifted the last two challenges to start on the seventh of their respective months. Regarding the order in which the diets done, except for the fact that the initial challenge was inspired directly by a client and the second by an upcoming trip to the United Kingdom, there was no specific logic for the order. Mostly, the choice of what diet to do next was based on how I felt the last week of the challenge before. Looking in retrospect now, I would risk saying that I gained momentum as the year went on, and discuss this in further detail in the text that follows.

This is a book about food, yet you will notice that there are no food pictures in the book. There is a reason for that. This is not meant to be a recipe book or even a health book. Although it is a book about food, I actually consider it to be more similar to a travel log. Keep in mind, I do love to cook and have learnt to photograph food, so I frequently posted pictures of the foods cooked and eaten throughout the year. You will easily find these in my Instagram (https://www.instagram.com/sofia.c.pereira/) account. The all tagged with #30daychallenge and then with further hashtags with the specific challenge of the month, so they should be easy to find. Mostly I cook without recipes, but am inspired by cooking and recipes from others, that then adapt to my tastes as well as to the ingredients currently around the house. So, if you see something you would like to eat and the recipe is not posted, send me an e-mail and I will be happy to help you out. I can tell you what is in it, mostly.

What about the food and drink challenges? How deep did I delve into each experience? The answers to those questions are obvious, I guess, by the existence of this book. I did not just impose specific eating limitations on myself for a month and then move on to the next one. As a scientist and a health coach, I have always loved to dig through the literature (scientific publications) and study the biological effects of different diets and lifestyles. Of course, this was even more so during this past year, where my interest was highly augmented by the personal aspect of experiencing certain symptoms or effects of certain diets. For clarity, the motivation of these experiments was not to lose weight or change my body shape. However, I have done some body shape metrics after each challenge, such as waist perimeter and weight. Also, compelled by many people annoying me about the effects of some of the regimes on my health, I did blood analysis after the ketogenic month and at the end of all the challenges. This data is sprinkled throughout specific sections as well as demonstrated in a summarized form in the appropriate sections at the end of the book. There is one thing that I must make very clear. This work is not intended to be a scientific publication or a therapeutic tool. Rather, it is a qualitative analysis of twelve food experiments, or thirty-day challenges, done consecutively over a one year period. Whatever opinions I have are my personal views and obviously influenced by my subjective feelings, and by no means meant to be objective "absolute truths". Regarding the scientific research used for the discussions, there are reference lists at the end of the chapters where they are cited.

The format of the book is simple and hopefully easy to read. Each experiment or thirty-day challenge is presented as a separate chapter and contains random entries within the thirty-day period. At the end of each section, there is a short paragraph with a conclusion as well as a list of pros and cons that I felt during that challenge. To give insight into the long-term influence of each specific limitation, I have also added an "in retrospect" paragraph or two at the end of each chapter, which was written in the few months following the completion of all twelve monthly challenges. These in retrospect sections, which are presented in italics, are meant to show the impact of specific limitations as well as how they are viewed in context of the whole. Also, I have asked my husband and kids a few questions about how these twelve months affected them and what they thought about it. Their wonderful words can be found in the final section, entitled "afterthoughts", which wraps up my experiments and hopefully ties up all loose ends.

Now let us focus on the most important part of this whole project, the reader… which is you. I really hope you connect with the book and that you look forward to reading it every time you pick it up. As I mentioned before, I have written and published a lot of science in scientific journals, and I have never worried about whether the reader was enjoying my writing. Now I worry. I want you to enjoy it and to be partially sad that it is over when you get to the end and read the final word. Not only do I hope you have fun reading this, I also hope that these twelve experiments are informative to you. Perhaps you have thought about trying a new diet. If that is the case, I think you may find the daily log of your diet choice interesting and perhaps helpful. One of the things I most became aware of during this past year was the lack of general knowledge of food intolerances, limitations or eating styles. Food culture is not a bad thing to be informed about. Furthermore, and more importantly, I would love if my experiences inspire you to try to explore your own food self. No matter what your background or profession, I believe that trying new healthy foods and going beyond your current eating habits only brings advantages.

There is little doubt that variety is important when it comes to what we eat. This is obvious by just thinking of a key phrase commonly used to promote healthy eating, "eat a rainbow every day". And this, of course, does not mean eating a handful of colorful candy daily. Rather, the rainbow reference means eating a wide variety of wholesome fresh foods, and mostly refers to the enormous diversity of colors in edible plants. A daily menu with a variety of plant foods provides us with all kinds of nutrients in their natural form, which builds us as well as feeds the symbiotic organisms that inhabit our gut. This incredibly complex population of bacteria and other living things (virus, fungus and archaea bacteria) play an extremely relevant role on our physical and mental health. Many studies have shown that the population of microorganisms (often referred to as the microbiome) in our guts is highly adaptable and responsive to what we eat, and that there are alterations in specific species in the guts of people with numerous diseases or pathologies. In general, species variability is a sign of health, and diverse species thrive on different foods. In sum, it is good for us to eat whole foods high in fiber, as it is precisely the fiber that we cannot digest that feeds microbiome and allows it to help our bodies (including our brains) stay healthy.

Enough of the health lesson, let us talk about food from a practical perspective. Trying new foods and recipes is not always easy, but it can be great fun if taken in stride. Also, as we expand our food repertoire and cooking comfort zone, successes such as great "quickly invented" recipes with what is available in the cupboard and fridge become more frequent. It is needless to say that great meals give us great pleasure. Considering that we eat every day many times a day, it is worth the investment to explore with foods. Of course, we must keep in mind when we try something completely new... it is never a good idea to wear brand new shoes for a ten-kilometer marathon. Also, new foods should be introduced gradually to see how our body reacts, with timing also being relevant. Although we may not deal well if we eat a bowl of whole grains just before we go for an intense workout, we could possibly feel great if we ate the same bowl and then went for a long slow hike. When it comes to our eating choices, we must be smart... but not forget that we tend to put our heads in front of our bodies and not the other way around. Yes, we should use our intelligent brains, but always listen to our bodies and follow instincts.

To conclude, I really hope you enjoy reading the log as I go through monthly regimes and that they serve to motivate you through your own food experiments, or inspire you to try some food challenges yourself. There is no doubt that self-imposed experiments and can be highly positive on a personal level, regardless of who you are or what you do. If you are a health professional or are close to someone with a food intolerance, these kinds of initiatives are a great way to walk the talk. Not only does living the experience ourselves allow us to feel what it is like to eat a certain way, it helps us better support others that are undergoing the same or similar regimes. Also, living it motivates greater involvement. The personal interest and deeper desire to do research and study further, in turn, allows us to better support our clients, family members, or friends that follow a food regime. Even if you are not a health professional, but you know someone who follows a specific eating style, many diets are associated with a certain type of lifestyle or philosophy, which is always interesting from a cultural point of view. Finally, another positive outcome of the food challenges, excluding the "no coffee" and "no alcohol" challenges which are health promoting just by themselves, all the rest increase knowledge and awareness regarding the consumption of processed foods. These are all good things, and I seriously hope you will decide to take on a challenge. In the end, you may be amazed by the huge amount of self-discipline that you actually do have, which translates into self-empowerment and often gives you the push to continue to explore your healthy self.

And now, here's is my log of a highly interesting year. Hope you enjoy it!

CHAPTER 1 – GLUTEN FREE

Three days ago, a client of mine mentioned that she was interested in trying to cut gluten from her diet to see if it helped her chronic stomach issues. After our talk, and thinking about the much-publicized gluten sensitivities and intolerances, I started to become interested in how I could best support my client through this change in eating. Looking at my own food choices, I concluded that I eat way too much foods made with wheat flour, especially bread. Whether because it's the easy choice or because I really do like it, a quick look-into my daily food intake made me realize that I am grabbing for bread at least three times a day. Sometimes it is just a chunk ripped off the loaf that is sitting in the bag on the counter, other times I make myself a sandwich or use bread as an accompaniment in a meal. Let me be clear, it's not that I have anything against bread… nor do I have any gluten sensitivity that I am aware of. I do, however, have something against lack of variety when it comes to my food choices. Also, maybe cutting out bread for a while will help me lose a couple of kilograms that seem to be very attached to my waistline for the last decade. All this together and I decided to see what happens if I completely cut out gluten from my diet for two weeks.

Day 1
I did not realize that gluten, an integral component of wheat and it's evolutionary relatives such as barley and rye, is everywhere! Today, I became acutely aware that this is not going to be easy, especially for an assumed flexitarian (which, by the way, simply means someone with no food restrictions)!

Day 2
Although I am already missing fluffy, elastic wheat bread, I am starting to enjoy the challenge. My stomach feels a bit different... similar to that feeling you get on an empty stomach. Funny, I find myself to always be slightly hungry, even after a good meal.

Day 4
Or is it? Last night, which was day three, I went to meet a friend in downtown Lisbon. After attending a lecture on male/female energy at the Instituto Macrobiótico de Portugal (Portuguese Macrobiotic Institute), we went for dinner at an Asian fusion noodle house. I ordered a noodle dish described on the menu as being prepared with buckwheat pasta. When dinner arrived, I found the noodles themselves to be surprisingly flexible and lacking the characteristic nutty buckwheat taste. I have to admit though, it was ten o'clock at night and I was starved, and ended up devouring the whole thing trying hard not to eat too fast. Afterwards, I asked the waitress how the noodles were made and quickly realized by the puzzled look on her face that she had no clue what I was asking. The conversation went something like this. I asked, "Could you please tell me what the pasta in my soup was made from?" And she responded, looking smug, "Wheat, and it's homemade." Then I said, "But it says on the menu that it was made from buckwheat, which is very different from wheat and has no gluten." To which she retorted "I only said it was made from wheat flour, I did not say it had gluten."
I felt my face getting hot while realizing this interaction was quickly

turning into a conversation not worth exploring. In the end, I left the restaurant irritated and feeling unresolved on whether I had eaten gluten or not. On the way home, I realized how difficult it must be to have serious issues with gluten, like for example to have gluten sensitivity or intolerance, as is the case for those with celiac disease. After getting home and about one hour after eating, I had loads of gases and felt bloated, but was it the gluten or some of the other salts and additives they tend to put in Asian food? I will never know but I did learn a big lesson, that if I am really going to do a serious experiment and cut out gluten completely, I must be more careful about what I put in my mouth. Regardless of whether my noodles were gluten free or not, today I'm craving bread and intend to walk to the health food store later to buy some gluten free flour variety or bread.

Day 8

I lasted one week, woohoo! Proud to be here! This is not an easy experiment for a bread fanatic, although I must admit it is getting easier. As I wrote in my last entry, which was on a Friday, I did go to the health food store to shop for gluten free bread, which was made with corn flour. Unfortunately, it looked absolutely disgusting and very similar to that horrible packaged white loaf breads that I haven't eaten since high school over thirty years back. Sadly, I toasted it and ate it accompanied by tea, and even more sadly, I enjoyed it. The positive outcome from this experience is that while eating my toast, I realized I needed to find an alternative… thank goodness that when it comes to what we put in our mouths, there are always alternatives! And so it was, alternatives were forged. Over the weekend, which corresponded to gluten free days five and six, I made all kinds of wholesome and yummy gluten free breads and other goodies. For baking, I used homemade whole rice and/or chickpea flour. What a pleasure to bake and to eat. The house smelt wonderful, and the kids loved everything I made! Saturday morning started off with chickpea and rice flour pancakes and then a trip to the health food store to buy psyllium husks for a rice flour/psyllium husk/milk bread recipe. Sunday morning, I baked a fresh loaf. My health coach's recipe, thank-you Patricia, made the best bread! Loved it then and am still enjoying it two days later.

Besides all the cooking and baking, do I feel different after one gluten free week? I think so. I feel like I have less of a belly and am "thinning out", probably because I tended to eat a fair bit of bread and am therefore just eating less. I am also enjoying the experience from an anthropological point of view; such as the options and lack of them when eating out; what to shop for and to cook; what pasta alternatives are there that serve as easy family dinner options, etc. At least one more week and then we'll see what I do. Maybe I will weigh myself tomorrow (which I haven't yet) so I can track any changes in weight. If I was asked right now whether I would repeat the experiment, my answer would be a resounding YES!

Day 9

I am hungry and in dire desire of some fluffy, flexible, crusty, chewy and wonderful smelling wheat bread from the bakery next door! Amazing how up and down this experiment has been… some days I think that this is exactly what I need and other days, like today- which is rainy and cold for Portuguese standards in May, I feel that I am insane to put myself through this torture. I still haven't weighed myself, so maybe that is the answer. Since I quit smoking almost two and a half years ago, and decided not to weigh myself for at least one year so as not to despair, I tend to forget to step on the balance and leave those metrics up to my less than yearly visits to the doctor. I guess now is the time, so I'm off to do that and then to exercise. Hopefully that will get my mind off gluten rich bread and pasta!

Back from doing a workout and then stepping on the balance, and the results were 61 kg in track pants and long sleeve t-shirt just after lunch. Although I am committed to re-weighing myself tomorrow morning before breakfast, this has been my normal weight for the last few years, and I would like to reduce it by a few kilograms.

Day 10

My morning weight in undies was 60.3 kg. Today I am making another gluten free bread loaf to take to my aunt who just got out of the hospital for knee surgery.

Day 13

One more gluten free weekend! I am extremely proud to have gotten through this last weekend, I have to admit… especially considering that we had a birthday dinner party with lots of very appetizing and undoubtedly delicious wheat based foods. Now I know why people that don't eat gluten are generally thinner. Without eating bread or cracker type appetizers, and with pasta and cakes for desert being off limits, it is much more difficult to over eat. I did make a great chickpea bread yesterday, so one good thing is that I now feel completely comfortable whipping up my own flour with seeds, whole grain rice, and various nuts or legumes in the food processor and baking up a bread.

Day 14

Today is the final day of the two-week long gluten free experiment and I seriously screwed up, I drank beers! Here goes what happened, full disclosure. A girlfriend of mine, who is going through a tough break up, dropped by for support and to vent and we ended up sitting at a bar on the beach and drinking beers! I completely forgot about my gluten free challenge, and only when happily downing my third small draft beer did I realize what I was doing. Within one hour, I felt like I swallowed an entire cow, a feeling that remained for the rest of the day. I am not sure if it was the gluten or the fact that I haven't touched beer in two weeks. I do feel bad about it, but decided to chalk it up to experience… like the coaching specialists say "look at your failures with curiosity".

On another note, I have decided to continue with this experiment for a while longer.

Day 20
Almost three weeks into this challenge and I am doing well and getting creative with gluten free cooking. Decided to extend the gluten free experiment for a full month. I did weigh in yesterday at minus 300 g and think I may be a bit thinner. The question remains whether it is it the gluten, or simply the fact that I am so limited in what I can eat. I don't know, but we will see what happens after the month. Also, I decided to do more food experiments as I find them really enriching from an anthropological point of view. With this in mind, I think I have already decided what the next experiment will be. Considering that I will be travelling a lot, and that I am a coffee addict, it seems to be a great time to go without coffee for one month. As always the case with our conscious decisions, there are many more reasons why this will come in handy, but those are to be disclosed in another chapter, the next chapter...

Day 24
Today, I feel like I have had enough of the gluten free, although I will hang in there for one more week. Can't wait to have some yum wheat bread in the morning and to eat a great pasta dish. To be honest, I think these desires mostly arise from being sick of having culinary limitations and not being able to eat things I enjoy. Like most people, I do not like to be told what to do. As I age, I notice that I am becoming increasingly anarchic and less and less into fitting into someone else's idea of reality. Ok, enough philosophizing... got to hang in there one more week!

Day 28
Counting down the days until there are no restrictions on what I eat. It's not the gluten free per se, I actually enjoy a lot of gluten free foods. It is just that I am sick of not being able to eat everything. On the other hand, I weighed myself today and I am down another 100 g. Also, I measured my waist circumference and it has reduced by 2 cm compared to the first day I weighed myself. I guess the

restrictions are doing something positive in that regard. In the end, I think this challenge has had many positive effects, such as the fact that I have learnt how to make different flours and breads without using the bread machine. Will it have long-term effects on my eating habits? Probably.

Day 30

Last gluten free day and I can't wait until it's over! It seems that I have reached the point that I am constantly feeling irritated by the limitation. I can see the positive side of the experience, but I am getting cravings for sugary stuff and believe that these are related to the fact that I can't have a slice of bread or a bowl of pasta. This week, I bought "semi unhealthy white flour" bagels, cream cheese and smoked salmon to enjoy on my day off. For breakfast tomorrow, I am really looking forward to digging my teeth into the gluten rich wheat flour bagels. I will accompany this with a large cup of piping hot coffee with milk, the last coffee breakfast for a while…

Conclusion

In the end, I am very glad that I did a gluten free month. From an experimental point of view, these 30 days were enriching in many ways. They definitely changed my all too frequent habit of eating bread based meals. Also, going gluten free pushed me to learn how to make breads and bake with different flours, such as chickpea, almond, oat and rice. As a result, and because it stopped being part of my daily routine, I think I will most likely eat less gluten in the future. The realization that gluten (from wheat or other gluten containing cereals such as spelt, barley, and rye) was everywhere was also an eye opener. It makes me question if we simply eat too much of it and therefore have become partially intolerant. We will see how my future relationship with this highly mediatized complex molecule present in wheats and their ancestors goes. For now and to wrap up this month, here are the positives and negatives as I see them.

Positives
- Weaned off the frequent daily (2-3 times a day, on average) bread meals or snacks.
- Explored with making different flours and baking various breads.
- Could not eat sugary cakes or baked goods in bakeries or when out for dinner.
- Lost 1 kg in 1 month, likely due to limitations.
- Lost 2 cm waist circumference.
- Had regular bowel and intestinal movements.
- Learnt about Psyllium husks.

Negatives
- Hate having food limitations.
- Parties and social gatherings were difficult.
- Felt gassy, especially in the first two weeks and probably due to adjustments to diet changes.
- Felt lack of energy, also especially the first two weeks and likely for the same reasons as above.
- Could not drink beer (except for screw up on day 14).
- Kids and husband complained that they miss pasta at mealtimes.
- Felt constantly hungry.

My day off

Woohoo, no limits! Enjoyed a bagel with cream cheese and smoked salmon this morning for breakfast, accompanied by a large cup of Dutch style coffee with milk. It tasted great! So far, no symptoms from having consumed wheat for the first time in a long time. We'll see how it goes, but I right now I am seriously looking forward to an ice-cold beer later on tonight!

In retrospect

More than an entire year has gone by since I did this challenge, and I am in awe reading about how difficult it was for me to go gluten-free for a month. Did it change how I eat? Yes, it has. I currently don't eat as much bread or pasta as I used to. In fact, my whole family eats less pasta, and what used to be a once a week dinner choice for us is currently probably closer to being a once a month option or less. But considering that many challenges were done after the gluten free month, I am finding it hard to pinpoint how this specific month changed my or our eating habits. I also enjoyed the realization that the decision to go on with consecutive food experiments only happened sometime halfway into this particular challenge, and it was definitely not to do them for a full year. Also, it is very cool to see that it was the only food experiment in which I cheated, and unconsciously or not, ate gluten twice throughout the month. On one hand, it shows that a it is what is part of our routines that really counts, and two isolated cheats do not take away from the validity of the year as long as it stays as that... two isolated cheats and not an excuse to give up and stop doing the challenge.

H. Sofia de Campos Pereira

CHAPTER 2 – COFFEE FREE

My new experiment is to go without coffee for a month. The reason I chose this challenge is somewhat similar to the reason for going gluten free, I know that I drink way too much coffee. Especially after having quit smoking two and a half years ago, I can easily drink three expressos in a day, sometimes straight up and sometimes with a drop of milk or milk foam. Thank goodness I don't like sugar in my coffee. Regarding my coffee addiction, I would like you to keep in mind that drinking multiple coffees in a day is quite a common practice in Portugal, where expressos often start the day and cap off every meal. Anyway, I am aware of the effects of coffee on me and the fact that it has become an all too frequent habit. That, taken together with the fact that I will be travelling for the next month to the land of tea (UK) for the world championships of grass ultimate, makes now the perfect time to go without my liquid gold for 30 days.

Day 1
The first thing I did on my first day without coffee was go to the neighborhood café, stand at the counter, and wait until they served me my perfect foamy expresso. As I was standing there, it sunk in… no coffee for this chick! Oh boy! I was grateful that the gluten free stint was done and bought bread, and then went home feeling like something was missing. The whole day I had a slight headache and

felt sleepy. We will see if I can go a whole month without my beloved "cafézinho".

The Portuguese, like me, characteristically love their coffee, it is part of our culture. As such, there are many ways to say coffee in Portugal. It's actually interesting that many of them don't even have the word coffee in them, such as "bica", which is the typical way to ask for an expresso in the Lisbon area, whereas in Porto it is "cimbalino". There is also "galão" (coffee with milk served in a tall glass), "meia de leite" (half coffee and half milk served in a shallow mug), "pingado" (the word means with a drop and is used to order an expresso with a touch of milk or some strong alcoholic beverage, for example Portuguese moonshine) and at least four more that I can think of (garoto, escaldado, curto, carioca). It is a much-loved bean in my small corner of the world.

Day 2

Still have a headache, still want a coffee, still not sure if I can do it

Day 3

No headache today, but still feeling a bit fuzzy and craving coffee. I'm slightly afraid that I will compensate my lack of coffee with junk food, as I am getting cravings for sweets. Oh, I must hold out and be strong.

Day 8

Finally, after a full week of struggling, a clear mind again and no more headache. I am glad to know that I can read, concentrate, assimilate, connect, create, think, focus and function without coffee! Thank goodness, as I do have some writing to do and I just hate fuzzy head focusing and writing. Feeling strong and healthy and still not eating much gluten, maximum one serving a day. And hopefully starting today, feeling energetic again!

Day 12

Patrick and I are off to London for ten days for the World Ultimate and Guts Championships (WUGC2016), and I hope it will not be too difficult not to drink coffee. The last few days, I feel like I have been eating a little too many sweets for my liking, and it worries me to think how I will compensate for the lack of coffee the following three weeks, which will be crazy. First, we are going to London for a few weeks to work with ERIC, which stands for Early Recognition is Critical, a non-for-profit organization that teaches the sport of ultimate as a vehicle for educating youth about cancer symptom awareness and to speak up when they feel something is wrong. I am really looking forward to that, and think it is an important cause. After London, we are coming back into Lisbon and immediately packing off to Meco to play and party at the 20th edition of the Bar do Peixe Beach Ultimate Frisbee tournament (BDP) for four days. With eleven games on soft beach and lots of late nights and parties over the four days, BDP is an endurance test or physical challenge in itself. Looking at things from a positive perspective, at least I won't be overdoing it on coffee, although truth be told I expect to be eating and drinking a fair bit of non-health promoting stuff for the next three weeks.

Day 18

It has been insanely busy in London and at the WUGC2016. Our ERIC booth is in the same tent as the bar, and since we often don't have a chance to leave the booth and go get food, we end up feeding mostly on beer during the day. If I could drink coffee, I would probably be overdoing it on that as well. Every day, I am amazed at how difficult it is not to cheat… especially at breakfast and while working at the booth where fresh coffee smell wafts in from the coffee stand nearby. I am often coming close to cheating, especially because I had forgotten how much I actually like crappy coffee with milk and sugar. In fact, back in my PhD days in Toronto, I did some of my best genetics work (complex classical genetics crosses in

Drosophila) with a huge cup of Tim Horton's coffee with double cream. But I haven't cheated, and thanks to English breakfast tea, have managed ok.

Day 30

Still coffee free. And it has been tough. This also means that I survived the first Bar do Peixe (BDP) without my critical and much needed morning (morning at BDP means 2 pm after a night of going to bed when the sun is already up) and after dinner expressos! Oh, I am just now having a brain fart... the lack of coffee may explain why I was so pooped and ended up struggling to keep my eyes open at the two of the four parties of the tournament. That makes me happy, as I prefer the lack of coffee reason to the option that I am just getting old, and therefore not able to enjoy myself at the parties because I am getting so sleepy. Well, it's done and I did it. One more challenge met! Proud to have succeeded and looking forward to the next one.

Conclusion

I am very happy to have gotten through this one, and it was much more difficult than I thought. At the beginning of the 30 days, I was surprised at how strong the physical symptoms of coffee withdrawal were. Especially the first week, when I felt stupid, fuzzy headed, tired and not functional. Thank goodness that the initial horrible phase was quick to pass, although it did make me realize how off quilter and addicted my body was.

Positives
- Weaned off an addiction.
- Managed to do what I said I would even thought it was hard, which is great for my ego.
- Will not drink 3-4 coffees a day anymore (I hope).
- Eventually got a clear functional mind back without the coffee (took one week).

Negatives
- I do not like limits!
- Had many sugar cravings.
- Found that not being able to use coffee as a recreational wake up drug after dinner party nights resulted in the night being less fun because I was sleepier.
- Weighed in at 61.4 Kg, which means i gained approximately 2 kg this month. However, this was more likely due to the crappy eating and drinking associated with travel than to the no coffee challenge itself.

My day off

Started the morning with one of my all-time favorite breakfasts, a piping hot and strong "galão", which is similar to a latte and served in a tall glass, and Portuguese rustic bread toasted with butter! Happy to be finished with this experiment, but also happy to have put a stop to my coffee addiction. Considering that the gluten free experiment did change how much bread I eat, evident as that many days now I don't even eat any bread, my target is to reduce my coffee intake. I hope to drink a maximum of two coffees a day from now on, and keep it to one except on special days. I am still undecided what my next challenge will be, which starts tomorrow!

In retrospect

I can only smile as I write this immediately after I come back from my second expresso of the day. One year later, and I am likely exactly where I was before I did this challenge as far as my coffee consumption is concerned. I probably drink two to three coffees a day, which means that my resolution to keep it to one or two a day did not hold out. I am aware of my "coffee-holic" tendencies, and often stop myself from walking to my friendly corner café and ordering a "cafézinho" every time I feel like it. Does my coffee consumption worry me? No, not at all. I feel great and healthy and would likely drink way less coffee if lived in a place that the coffee wasn't so good and cheap (I pay 65 cents per expresso at the café at the corner). My relationship with coffee and current coffee consumption are completely contrary to the long-term effects of "weaning off an addiction" from bread that I felt and still feel after the first gluten free challenge. Going without gluten for a month has made an impact on me to this day, I eat less bread than I used to.

CHAPTER 3 – OVO-LACTO VEGETARIAN

After much pondering over the last 24 hours about what challenge to do next, I have decided that my third food exploration experiment is to not eat meat or fish for the next month. Happily, I have company this time. As soon as I announced the decision to not eat animal flesh, my daughter Sara told me she is going to join me. Let's see how this goes, but somehow, I think it will be the easiest challenge so far.

Day 2
So far, nothing feels different or out of the normal. Likely I think this due to this eating style, consisting of various dairy products, eggs and a lot of plant based foods, being very similar to how I normally eat. This evening should be interesting. We are going downtown into Lisbon to have dinner while watching Portugal play Wales in the EURO semi-final soccer game. Portugal is not the best place for nutritionally challenged people to eat out, and I wonder if it's going to be difficult to get a good dinner without meat or fish.

Day 3
I woke up feeling sick today with a summer flu. Considering the physical demands of the last few weeks, including the crazy time in London followed by the four-day tournament and associated parties, I am not surprised. Summer flu, quick to come, quick to go. And I

am still smiling about last night, which turned out to be a great night in Lisbon, starting off with dinner in a cool Portuguese restaurant with an old friend from Canada and then celebrating a victory for Portugal (2-0) against Wales in a large city square (Terreiro do Paço) full of happy Portuguese people and tourists. Interesting how difficult it was to eat a healthy meal without animal meat. Luckily, the restaurant served "fish from the orchard", a typical Portuguese tempura like dish made with battered and fried green beans. Then there was salad and soup, and not many more options. Oh, and Sara is already off the diet. She found the restrictions to be too inconvenient with all the summer barbeques. Plus, she felt rude not eating whatever was being served by her friend's parents when at friend's houses for a meal. I understand and know just how she feels, food restrictions can be very anti-social.

.

Day 7

Today marks the day that I am one week into this challenge and I feel that it is getting tougher. Funny thing is that I think my sub-conscious mind is telling me something through my dreams. Yesterday, Patrick and I watched the EURO final against France in a Pizza place (where I dined on a salad and drank cider) and afterwards celebrated Portugal becoming European soccer champions on the streets of downtown Lisbon. We got home late, happy and tired, so I fell asleep fast and deep. Overnight, I dreamt about eating raw, live, swimming fish. This morning, the first thing that went through my mind when I woke up was that I wanted to eat any kind of animal. To be honest, I am not particularly enjoying this experiment and actually feel a bit physically and mentally weak after just one week. Amazing, especially considering that I don't eat that much meat normally and only one week has gone by. If I try to forget my food desires by pushing myself physically and working out, the lack of strength and energy just gets worse, like for example this morning when I went running. One thing is for sure, I am not going to try to go vegan for a full month. In fact, I am right now really looking forward to the paleolithic diet – give me meat!

Day 10

I still have not eaten any animal flesh and am happy to say that my crazy cravings and weird graphic dreams about eating live animals have died down a bit. Something happened this morning that I have never experienced before, I woke up with cramps in the calf muscles of both my legs. I think it is likely to be related to not eating meats, as is the weakness in my muscles that I feel since a week into this challenge, especially if I run up the stairs or push my body to do something physically more strenuous for more than a few minutes. I am right now slightly worried and curious about how it will go tonight at a dinner party. Considering that there will be a set menu, I am curious about whether there will be healthy options. Also, will I come across as rude because I don't eat what is offered to me?

Regarding the logistics of what foods to eat, I don't find it too difficult to be an ovo-lacto vegetarian when I eat at home, where the possibilities are endless. I normally don't eat much meat anyway, on average red meat about once a week, chicken once or twice a week and ditto for fish. But going to other people's homes for dinner or eating out at restaurants is a whole new ballgame. It can be tricky not to be that horrible guest that snubs her nose at what is offered. For the sake of transparency, which I ardently believe in, I feel the need to write here that I am going to take 360 mg fish oil tabs for Omega-3 fatty acid, in the hope of offsetting the fatigue and muscle tiredness that has set in. Hopefully it will help. I can't believe that there are still twenty days to go. In the end, this is a serious exercise in self-discipline.

Day 14

I survived another weekend without eating flesh, and this one was not an easy one. Once again, my immediate family of four was invited to a family dinner party in a restaurant, to celebrate the 18th birthday of my cousin's and close friend's daughter. At the party, most of the healthy options on the pre-chosen menu consisted of some type of sea carcass, which means that I drank much more that I ate. Although I had a load of fun celebrating the birthday of someone who is dear and close to me and my family, the self-imposed eating limits were not easy, nor was keeping away from some amazing looking and probably very delicious seafood. To add insult to injury, I felt rude politely and sheepishly turning foods away or leaving them on my plate. By the end of the night, and because there was so little that I could eat and gin and tonics don't have animal protein, I ended up drinking way too much.

The second food related difficulty this past weekend was brought on by a beach ultimate league day with four games, which was held in a gorgeous beach 40 km south of Lisbon. Considering that the party was the night before, I didn't have time to prepare food to take to the beach, and the beach restaurant had a very limited menu of healthy options for my current eating regime. Bread with crappy cheese accompanied by chips did not seem the least bit appetizing compared to their famous squid dishes. That is my biggest beef (no pun intended) with food limitations, they do not favor the healthy option, especially when away from home.

On a more positive note, and taking into account how physically weak I have been feeling lately, I was happy to have been able to play decently and to feel physically strong the entire beach ultimate league day. Sadly, as if often the case after doing a lot of sports, I craved red meat. Bearing in mind the current limitations, spicy Indian vegetarian food turned out to be a good alternative, although Patrick and I had a "first" when it comes to the definition of hot-spicy food. We arrived at the restaurant late after the games, around 10:30 pm on a Sunday night, and were the only costumers there. We were both afraid the kitchen would be closed, and were happy to be led to a table with the promise of a late dinner.

Patrick and I both love hot-spicy Indian food, and asked for a spicy vegetarian dish. However, the wonderful smelling curry they served us was so spicy that, for the first time in our lives, we just could not eat it. Not even with a load of basmati rice. I have since thought of the possibility that the waiters were unhappy to have to serve us so late, and therefore tried to kill us with spice. Earlier this evening for dinner, I used the leftovers of the vegetarian spicy dish that I brought home in a takeaway container, added chickpeas, more vegetables and a can of coconut milk. Even after such a large dilution, although edible and enjoyed by all, we still found the curry to be just slightly too spicy. And this for a family that eats a lot of spice.

Day 20

One more week gone by as an ovo-lacto vegetarian and holding on strong to my willpower not to cheat, even though I am desperately missing eating animal flesh. Truth be told, I feel that the weakness in my body and the overwhelming desire to eat meat or fish is a telltale sign that this regime is making me deficient in some vitamins and minerals. Once again looking towards solutions, I am aware that only now am I starting to know how to eat within this self-imposed limitation. I had a very good and satisfying vegetarian meal two nights ago at a vegetarian restaurant in Lisbon. After proper appetizers and a main course of mystic kebob with tofu, pineapple and seitan, I actually felt full for hours and went to bed without a hole in my stomach. This experience has made me think that perhaps I have to adjust how I cook and eat as a vegetarian, and am now looking forward to a special dinner at a vegetarian restaurant for my birthday in a couple of days. On the other hand, I am counting down the days to being able to eat some awesome Portuguese grilled fish.

Day 22

Tomorrow is my 51st birthday, holy cow! How did fifty two years go by? Well, I am happy to be where I am, and now onto more important things, food without meats. Last night while grocery shopping, I actually made sure to buy good protein-rich meat alternatives to cook with, such as seitan, tofu and quinoa. Today I made a great lunch, consisting of oven baked sweet potatoes, grilled seitan accompanied red pepper/red cabbage coleslaw. Feeling full and happy and ready to watch the second episode of season six of Game of Thrones. Funny how my mood changes when I am not feeling nutrient-deficient... maybe I am finally getting the hang of this vegetarian thing.

Day 27

Still hanging in there. Also, I am finally finding it easier not to compensate the lack of animal meat by eating too many eggs, or too much cheese, yogurt and nuts. On my birthday (July twenty-seventh), Patrick, the two kids and I went to a great vegetarian restaurant in Cascais called House of Wonders. I loved the food and the minty lemonade and would definitely go back there. Maybe with my daughter, who also adores to go out for lunch. Other than the few specialized vegetarian or vegan restaurants, Portugal is not easy for those who don't eat meat. So although my meal options at home have changed to fit the ovo-lacto vegetarian lifestyle, it is still extremely difficult to find wholesome options in traditional Portuguese restaurants. We went to spend a day with friends by the coast in Peniche a couple of days ago, where the fresh fish and seafood is just amazing. At a sea-side restaurant, I had to contend myself with vegetable soup for lunch and a greasy canned mushroom omelet for dinner. Not my first choices for sure, especially watching my husband and friends dig into a beautifully prepared dish of fresh scallops. Anyway, this adventure is almost done. For the sake of consistency, today I have decided that the fourth of every month will be my day off and the fifth day of each month the start of a new experiment.

Day 28

Last night after a great game of disc with my daughter's friends, we had dinner at home with six people, which included one of her friends and one of my friends. The dinner menu consisted of readily prepared vegetarian burgers and spinach sticks baked in the oven with homemade mashed potatoes and endive. This was the first time we are eating previously prepared foods in our house in a long time… which brings me to my next challenge, which will start in four days: no processed foods for a month.

Day 30

Final day as an ovo-lacto vegetarian and feeling ready to move on to the next challenge. Weighed in this morning at 59.9 Kg.

Conclusion

What an experience this month was, and considering that this eating style is not so different from my regular one, it was much tougher than I expected. Perhaps because it is the third month in a row where I impose a food limitations on myself or perhaps because of the longer-term effects of not eating animal flesh, I felt large differences in how I felt physically this month. Also, it took at least two weeks for me to sense that I had finally gotten the hang of how to eat this way without overdoing it on things that I already ate, such as milk, eggs, and cheese. This, of course, meant introducing things that I did not previously belong in my regular diet, such as seitan, tofu, and husks/seeds.

In general, I do not think I would ever chose this type of diet, and believe that with my current lifestyle, it limits the choices of what to eat and often forces me to eat the unhealthy option (such as a gin and tonic). I also believe that the lack of nutrients exclusively present in animal flesh, such as creatine and EPA and DHA Omega fats, resulted in me feeling weaker and less energetic. The biggest positive outcome of this month for me is the fact that this is the third food experiment that I complete, and after three months I feel a huge gain in self-discipline and self-trust. Can't wait to see how this whole adventure develops.

Positives

- One more time, I managed to do what I promised myself I would even thought it was not easy.
- I learnt more about cooking with legumes and quinoa as well as other vegetarian protein options such as seitan and tofu.
- I learnt what it means to eat this way and therefore will be able to better support my clients who chose this eating style.
- I realized the importance of animal protein in my diet, especially fish.
- Lost 1.5 Kg in one month without going hungry (mind you, I had 1 kg extra at the beginning of the month from the London trip).

Negatives

- Once again, I do not like having food limits and believe they often lead to choices that are not health promoting.
- The limits led to a tendency of overdoing it on starchy or unhealthy sugary foods.
- Felt serious muscle weakness and woke up in the middle of the night with leg cramps, which had never happened to me before except in the late stages of my pregnancies. These effects were mostly felt in the first two weeks.
- Got the flu, which may be completely unrelated.

My day off

Oh what a treat... I had a fantastic lunch out with my favorite three people (husband and kids, in case you're wondering) at a great seafood place called Eduardinhos, in Carcavelos. Plenty of seafood including octopus salad and fresh oysters... not bad choices for the first flesh I bite into in a month! Feeling great and ready for a new challenge, which starts tomorrow!

In retrospect

The third adventure in this journey was a surprisingly interesting one for me. Regarding the food limitation, I was not expecting it to be so difficult not to eat meat and fish, and was surprised by my instinctual need for animal flesh, including thoughts of eating live fish while swimming in the ocean or biting into live cows. It was so bizarre and odd that the mental images of the memories are still vivid in my mind. For example, while swimming with my son at the beach in front of our house and looking down in the clear water, I would imagine myself diving down to the small fish swimming beneath me, opening my mouth wide, and swallowing live fish… like a whale. These "I need flesh!" instincts often brought to mind a friend from graduate school, and how I could finally relate to him. Back then, I used to get shocked when he would tell us that the first thing that went through his mind when looking at a field of grazing cows was, "Dinner!".

Besides the specifics of ovo-lacto vegetarian month, some interesting things also came up while reading over and editing this third chapter. One is that I now realize that the whole year was not pre-planned at all. What I mean is that after three months of food challenges, I had no clue how or where this journey would end up. This is clear by reading over what I wrote about vegan, namely that I could never do it. What I like about this lack of pre-planning is that it shows that I must have enjoyed the process to keep doing it, as well as that it was the process itself that pushed things forward. It gives me a huge amount of satisfaction to see in practice what I constantly preach, that the result is part of the process.

Speaking of process, it was also sticking with the plan that eventually, after a couple of weeks, started to have an effect on the types of foods used at home to cook with and eat. Things take time, and if we are patient and persistent, change does occur. For the sake of completion, I must mention that this is one of the few times I got sick and felt weak throughout the food challenges year.

Keeping in mind that it may be purely coincidental, I also got quite sick and felt extremely during the vegan month. Would I do this regime voluntarily? No, I would not. I thought about it while enjoying that wonderful fresh seafood meal with my family on my day off and many times since. I never want to deprive myself of fresh fish, seafood or organic chicken, pork or beef. In my current life, where I live, activity level, etcetera, I believe that the best healthy option for me is to be a flexitarian. But I am glad I did it, I learnt a lot and it was undoubtedly an important part of my progress and food learning curve.

To conclude this chapter, I would like to share with you the difficulties that I am having as an author and editor. At a dinner party recently, and while discussing the possibility of this book being read by someone else besides me with some friends, a lot of interesting things came up. I have no idea what interests you, and tonight was important for me to get others feedback. For example, my cousin and close friend mentioned that it would be interesting to read about how the different experiments affected or changed the way we eat at home. And in fact, the challenges had a huge impact on what we eat. More specifically looking back on this particular month, which at the time was so difficult for me, I realize how much the ovo-lacto vegetarian widened the ingredients commonly found in our fridge and pantry as well as the types of meals we feel happy and comfortable cooking. Considering that almost a year has passed, I am happy to announce that these changes have undoubtedly enriched my and my family's experience with food.

CHAPTER 4 – WHOLE FOODS

My fourth food experiment is to not eat any processed foods for one month! What this means is that I can eat anything that has not been altered by human intervention since it was collected, and I can prepare it how I wish! Off limits are pasta, white flour, sugars, refined grains, any processed meats, sugars, and so on. I will have to read labels carefully. What I can eat includes natural milk, yogurt, and other dairy products, eggs, meats, fruits, vegies, and all other natural whole foods. Regarding alcohol, only naturally fermented alcoholic drinks without additives such as organic wine and beer are allowed. I am looking forward to this one, and actually believe that will be the easiest challenge to do so far, because I can eat any type of food. In fact, my prediction is that although this will be the least difficult challenge, it will be the one with the most impact on my body and how I feel, for the better of course. Today I weigh in at 59.9 kg and have a circumference around my belly button of 87 cm. I am curious to see how eating whole foods for 30 days will influence those parameters. Right now, I feel generally physically good, apart from sore and cramping muscles which may be due to lack of creatine since I haven't eaten any red meat for over a month. That will be quickly taken care of now, as I am off to walk to the butcher in the village to shop for a nice steak for dinner tonight.

Day 4

Day four on whole foods and I haven't felt the need to write as much, probably because I am just loving this food experiment! Finally, I don't feel limited in what I can eat! Partially because of my education as a biologist and health coach, I have a very clear knowledge of what whole foods are, and to the honest, the choices are endless! I have even made some yummy deserts, including a pudding with passion fruit and cream which was divine, or a fresh tangy raspberry, lemon, mint and chia seed sorbet.

Over the last couple of days, I have eaten at least one meal a day consisting of animal protein, including two red meat meals. The physical weakness I felt from not eating meat is gone, so I can exercise intensely again without getting all cramped up. Also, if we want to get into the details of physiological body functions, my intestines are working better than they have ever done before... one big happy dump in the morning... regular, satisfying, perfect! My period, which is usually extremely regular, was one week late and finally came on in full force. I am not sure if this unusual irregularity is due to not eating meat for a month or if it is simply attributable to normal pre-menopausal symptoms of a 51-year-old.

Day 10

Still going strong on whole foods, although I have had a few cravings for sweets or cool mixed cocktail drinks such as gin and tonic. Especially yesterday, Patrick and I walked to beach ultimate practice and there was a crepe maker on the boardwalk just as we were arriving. Patrick had a Nutella crepe that looked and smelled absolutely heavenly. Even with tough moments such as those, this is by far the most pleasant of the four food experiments. And, since I can now make whatever I want to eat as long as it's not processed, it has brought back my love for cooking and desire to try new meals. Another advantage of this regime is that although it can be difficult to eat out of the house, there are always options such as grilled meat or fish with lemon juice. The thing I miss the most is pasta... maybe

I will have to make it myself from whole durum wheat one of these days. So far, the biggest difficulty in my diet this month comes from the fact that I cannot eat any bread that is sold in the bakery close to home, which means that I eat almost no bread (again). All in all, I am very much enjoying this challenge and starting to be afraid to move on to the next one, where there will be restrictions on things I love to eat once again.

Day 20

My family of four, including me of course, is off for a small holiday in the south of Portugal and I am still going strong on whole foods. It has been great to see how much support I am getting from friends and family on this challenge, which I still think is the easiest one so far. As far as my three homies go, it is fantastic to see them reading labels and ingredient lists, with genuine interest about what is in foods and how to make choices based on what I can eat as well. For our holiday, we have rented a house in the Algarve for an extended weekend, which means we can cook our own whole foods based yummy dinners. So, we made a menu and went shopping together, and it was great to see the awareness of what is whole foods in the kids. Considering how much junk and processed food is out there, it satisfies me to know that my kids can make the choice from a position of knowledge.

Another positive aspect of this challenge is that I have learnt and really enjoyed making my own condiments with wholesome ingredients, especially mayonnaise (with added garlic or without), which everyone just loves. I guess the reason I haven't written much is because I am not finding this challenge to be so difficult and therefore feel very little need to vent. On the other hand, I am not losing weight at the rate I thought I would. This may be due to the fact that I am working out regularly and therefore hopefully gaining muscle mass. Also, I can eat a lot of different high calorie foods, such as nuts, that I love. As the weeks go by, I must admit that I am starting to get cravings for sugary stuff… especially when I go to the nearby café, *A Merenda*, where the "pasteis de nata" (Portuguese cream pastries) are absolutely delicious.

Day 23

I am now on holiday with the family in a country home close to Tavira in the Algarve. Loving the long days on the beach and the late nights of home cooked whole food meals and games with the family. Patrick and I decided to do a "no alcohol" holiday, so no white wine or beer but rather lots of cold water and yummy foods. Happily for me, there are two ice-cream houses in Tavira with organic ice-cream (no gluten, lactose, sugar or additives). There is nothing better than enjoying a fresh tasty treat late afternoon while still salty from the beach with my family – no cone though!

Day 30

Wow, Patrick and I married twenty three years ago today! I am sort of amazed at how happy and in love with each other we still are! But now back to the whole foods experiment at hand, I can't believe it is the last day of the 30 day whole foods challenge. I am afraid of all the ones that are to come, and have no doubt that they will be much tougher for me to complete. And even though I really enjoyed this month, I am most proud that I have managed to go 30 days without any refined sugar such as cookies, cakes and chocolate! This is an amazing feat for a sweet tooth such as myself. My guilty pleasure has been fried potatoes. Once more for the sake of transparency, there are some things that I have eaten this month that strictly speaking may not be considered a whole food: vegetable oils (olive oil, coconut oil), wine and beer (only the good stuff, made from fermented grapes or cereals, respectively), table salt (I only use pure sea salt in my cooking, but I have eaten grilled fish and/or meat as well as salads away from home), chips where the ingredients are exclusively potatoes and olive oil. I have chosen to include these as whole foods as long as there were no additives or conservatives. Tomorrow, I will weigh myself and measure my waist before indulging in a sugary treat made from condensed milk, Greek yogurt, and passion fruit that I just prepared and put in the fridge to solidify.

Conclusion

One more month and one more food experiment accomplished. Although, this one was nowhere near as challenging as the previous ones or, I am sure, the ones that are to come. In general, I loved eating whole foods. Furthermore, unlike with the gluten free or the vegetarian challenge, I felt that I always had an option of something to eat this last month. This may partially explain the result of my weigh in this morning, which showed my current weight to be at 59.7 Kg, meaning that I lost a measly 200 g in one month without processed sugars or flours. On the other hand, my waist circumference measured at 85 cm, which is 2 cm less than when I started the whole foods challenge. Considering that I have been on holiday and have not been playing or practicing ultimate in the last few weeks, this is a positive outcome.

Regarding what it felt like to eat exclusively whole foods, the truth is that the simple fact that I could eat from any food group or family (meat, dairy, fish, vegetables, fruit, whole grains, legumes, fermented foods) stimulated mine and Patrick's love for cooking. Which means that we both spent a lot of time in the kitchen these last 30 days, and invented fantastic meals! Since I am a sweet tooth and get sweet cravings, I regularly ate honey, which I sometimes poured over nuts and oats for a treat. Also, I feel I should mention that the tiredness and cramping that was so many times present in the last challenge was gone by the first week of this current challenge. My menstrual cycle is regular again, and I feel strong and energized physically and mentally. As far as my body and health are concerned, I am now convinced that I need to eat meat or fish to feel my best. Up to now, this was my favorite challenge by a long shot. I am not looking forward to having food limits again.

Positives

- I did not eat any sugary stuff that I love and did not cheat any time throughout this month (Nutella crepe was tough).
- Learnt a lot about certain foods I thought were whole foods and in fact are not, such as many cheeses (some are less than 50% milk and have starches such as potato starch added), creams (same as cheese), coconut milk, canned fruits, etc. Reading labels is incredibly important.
- The whole family learnt to read ingredient lists and to discern what is a whole food and what can be considered processed or refined.
- I got to seriously appreciate the interest and support that my family and friends are giving me throughout the challenges. In fact, decided during this challenge that I was going to ask my three homies that live with me to eventually write up a small summary about this experience from their perspective.
- Significantly expanded my capacity for quickly putting together whole food snacks and meals to go, especially picnics for full days on the beach.
- Lost 2 cm waist circumference and 200 g.

Negatives

- Cutting out sugars and other processed foods did not result in as much difference in my body as I thought it would, perhaps due to less physical activity than usual and the fact that we went on a holiday.
- I probably ate too much good quality cheese as a guilty pleasure.
- Got some serious sugar cravings, especially towards the end of the month.
- Sometimes it was difficult on my family to constantly be forced to eat whole grains instead or white flour products such as pasta, rice or bread.

My day off

Today, I satisfied my humongous desire for high quality Italian ice-cream, which has been off limits due to added sugars. Went to my absolute favored gelato place, called Santini, where they make the best fruit and nut gelatos. Oh so yum... huge cone, three flavors, heavenly!

In retrospect

Whenever people ask me which was my favorite of the 12 challenges, this one immediately comes to mind. Not surprisingly, really, as I could basically eat anything I felt like as long as it did not have processed or refined ingredients. In retrospect, whole foods was by far the easiest of the twelve months, as evidenced by the lack of frustrated and unhappy entries in my log. Partially, this can be attributable to the time of year being August, which means the kids had no school and we had some time away as a family on holidays. Due to my limitations eating out, most of our meals were made and eaten at home, or prepared at home and then taken to the beach. I must, however, mention that we went to an amazing grilled fish smorgasbord in Tavira, where I ate so much fresh grilled fish that I could hardly walk afterwards. Truly amazing! Another highly positive outcome of this month was the desire to go completely clean on our holidays in the South of Portugal, which means that we did not drink alcohol or relish in any other recreational drugs, including sugar. Happily, both Patrick and I didn't miss indulging at all!

CHAPTER 5 – DAIRY FREE

On to challenge number five… no dairy for one month! The reasons I decided to do this challenge are manifold. I had initially thought to go alcohol free for 30 days after the positive experience with the alcohol-free days on holidays last month. However, I am going to Holland for my brother in law's 50th birthday, and while talking to my mother in law about the possibility of being alcohol free while visiting, she wisely suggested that I take on a different challenge in order to be able to cheer my brother in law at his birthday bash. On top of that, I am very much aware of the absurd amounts of cheese and yogurt I ate in the last month when doing the whole foods challenge. Third and last, I think this is a valid challenge considering I will be in Holland for over a week and will have to curb devouring amazing Dutch Cheese, quark, and "vla" (a tasty milk based Dutch pudding). To be honest, I think this challenge is going to be very difficult to stick to.

Day 1
I just finished eating a soy yogurt with a slice of quinoa bread and some black berry jam and it was not as bad as I thought it would be. Although I must admit that the whole processing required to get yogurt from soy beans kind of freaks me out. But I did look carefully at the ingredient list, and the ingredients themselves for the natural

soy yogurt seemed ok. There must have been at least two times today that I opened the fridge and stared at the cheese. It almost made me cry. I do hope to lose some weight this month and therefore make the sacrifice worth it!

Day 3

Today I decided to treat myself to some high-gluten, fluffy, fresh bread from the bakery at the corner. I haven't had any in over one month and I really felt like a big fat sandwich. And so I walked over to the local bakery and asked to see the ingredient list for their approximately fifteen different kinds of breads, including carob, rye, whole wheat, spelt, corn, seeds, etcetera. Sadly, they ALL contained dairy in the form of milk powder! There were two that are dairy free on their list, but I have never actually seen them for sale! Walking a bit further to the supermarket at the village, I did find some dairy free whole wheat bread and had a prosciutto sandwich that tasted most awesome! So far, I am not having as hard a time as I thought I would without dairy. I found some oat milk that I enjoy putting in smoothies and oatmeal, and although I often want to eat cheese and butter, it's not that bad. Maybe after five months of challenges, I'm getting used to having self-imposed limits on what I eat. On another note, I do have some symptoms that may or may not be related to this challenge. For example, my knees hurt yesterday when I was running around on the sand at beach ultimate practice. Also, after having completely regular intestines for months, I am slightly constipated. Thinking further about this, it is more likely that my intestines are reacting to my going off whole foods and to the re-introduction of crappy preservatives, sugars and additives into my diet again.

Day 7

Admittedly and sadly, I am desperately craving milk products, especially butter and cheese. In fact, I had one of the worse craving days yesterday in a long time, which never ends up well. Started right in the morning eating coconut/egg/sugar cookies, had meat and a beer for lunch, gnocchi for dinner and then a whole pack of milk free cookies at night. Needless to say, my belly is not doing very well this morning. Also, although I decidedly do not like soy yogurt or milk, I did try rice-milk that is not bad even though I prefer the oat, almond, or coconut milk.

Day 13

Oh my god this is so tough! I have been in Holland for three days to celebrate my brother in law's 50th birthday and I am surrounded by amazing, appetizing, beautiful and oh-so-tasty high-quality dairy products! Throughout the five months of food challenges, I have never been so close to cheating as I am right now. But I knew this was going to be a challenge, especially because I just adore cheese and yogurt and Holland has the best cheeses and yogurts in the world! Of course, the little devil on my shoulder is constantly whispering in my ear. He seems to be insisting endlessly and saying, "eat whatever you want. Nobody cares about your stupid food challenges." And, "Why are you doing this anyway?" But I can hold strong... even if it's just for me and my self-discipline and self-trust! Interesting that I cannot find any oat milk in Holland, and bought coconut-rice milk instead. Also, I have forgotten to mention what a weakling I have become when it comes to alcohol... one glass of wine or one beer and I am spinning! This is a large difference from my pound-them-back with the boys days! Since we have been here in Holland, I do have one alcoholic beverage every day, which I thoroughly enjoy. Later on tonight is my brother in law's 50th birthday celebration, so let's see how much I drink and party at his hippie themed party.

Day 22

Not eating dairy while in Holland for a week turned out to be an extreme challenge, not only to my discipline but also to my patience. Especially because it was very clear to me that Dutch dairy foods were, by far, often the best choice of food as far as quality and health goes. Regarding the strong anti-dairy movement currently in the press and advocated by many health professionals, as far as I see it the Dutch are the perfect example of the wonderful benefits of healthy wholesome dairy. They are generally a very healthy and robust population, and, although I had never noticed before and was really interested to see, the Dutch eat a load of dairy.

I can think of many examples of situations throughout my stay in Holland that show how much dairy the Dutch eat. Perhaps because of their tendency to eat sandwiches and snacks all day long and have only one hot meal for dinner, it seems to me that dairy is often an opted for food choice in Holland. One afternoon in Patrick's mom hometown, Patrick and I went for lunch with his mom at a healthy sandwich place. It was cool to see that there was only one dairy free option on the entire menu, a humus and grilled vegetable sandwich, which I chose by default and was actually very good. Even on our last night there, dinner was white wine and wonderful finger foods, where the big star was a plate of amazing Dutch cheeses!

To add to these difficult to stay away from dairy experiences in the Netherlands, this last weekend we had a wedding back here in Portugal, and boy did I suffer. Most appetizers had some cheese or cream in them, as did the soup, and over 90% of the deserts. To add insult to injury, I had to avoid the richest and most appetizing cheese table loaded with wonderful, stinky, Portuguese cheeses. Although I am proud to say that I have still have not cheated, I must confess to something which I think is sort of disgusting: I bought butter flavored vegetable spread to put on toast and devoured a couple of slathered toasted slices of bread. Yum and yuck! One of the things I tell my clients not to use is margarine or vegetable spreads, as they are highly processed unnatural foods. But oh well, a little bad is good, as in the end it is what you do 80-90% of the time that counts.

Day 29

Thank goodness that I am almost at the end of this dairy free month.

At this point, I am seriously looking forward to digging my teeth into some old Dutch cheeses that we brought back from Holland. I have to admit, the last few days have been a bit of a debauchery when it comes to eating. I bought a large loaf of white "Alentejano" bread, which is like a rustic sower dough bread and is made simply from wheat, salt, water and yeast. Over the past couple of days, I have been ridiculously feasting on toast or soup with bread cubes. This kind of behavior is no longer normal for me. Also, while hanging out on the couch and watching TV after dinner, Patrick and I have been attacking the licorice that we brought back from Holland. Last week I had lost some weight and was happy with how things were going, especially because I have been practicing disc and working out regularly again... but I have a feeling that this week has been my disgrace. Oh well, that is life, no progress is linear.

Conclusion

This challenge was extremely tough for me, especially because of our trip to Holland. Admittedly, I have never been as close to cheating as I have during the last month, and often questioned why I am putting myself through these limitations. At the worst times, the monkeys in my head tell me that I am undergoing self-imposed suffering for no reason and should eat whatever I want. Of course, logically I know that the challenges are a good experience, even if in the end, they are just an exercise in self-discipline. Do I feel differently after not eating dairy for 30 days? Not really. Did it make a huge impact on my diet? Yes! Whereas I often ate a piece of cheese and some nuts when I was hungry, I couldn't... and I missed it terribly. I also missed butter a lot... and not only putting it on toast, but also for cooking. Regarding my weight, I gained 0.5 kg this month (60.2 kg) and 1 cm in waist circumference (86 cm). This may be simply because I have been overdoing it on crap food the last week, since for the last days I have not been making the healthiest choices and have been eating too much white Portuguese bread and cereal with oat milk. Regarding my other body parameters, such as intestinal functioning, menstrual cycle, and sleep, everything appears to be in perfect functioning order.

Positives
- Again, I did not cheat even though it was very difficult, especially while in Holland.
- This month was an educational experience regarding how much of what we eat has "hidden" dairy, including most baked goods and cereals.
- Found that things can be quite tasty without cheese, especially vegetable omelets, pasta and Mexican foods.
- Enjoyed trying different vegetable milks and spreads. Particularly enjoyed oat milk, although I found it a bit too sweet.
- Expanded my cooking with nuts, seeds, and seaweed to make up for the lack of cheese in my recipes.
- Found breakfast alternatives for milk based foods such as smoothie bowls and soft-boiled eggs.
- In general, did not go hungry as there was always a dairy free alternative.
- Maintained excellent energy levels throughout the month.

Negatives
- Missed eating cheese, butter, and yogurt terribly.
- Got some serious sugar and white bread cravings and gave in to these way too often.
- May have gained a bit of weight (although 0.5 kg is not really a gain) and 1 cm on my waist.
- Found it sad to say no to some amazing dairy foods, such as high-quality Dutch cheeses, creamy soups, desserts, etc.

My day off
Today, on my day off, I started the day with whole foods nut and date bread and a slice of cheese accompanied by a tall glass of cold

milk. Later in the day, Patrick and I ate a "pastel de nata" each (wonderful Portuguese cream pastry) with a "dropped" coffee (expresso with a drop of milk) before going for a workout. Also, I ate some great cheeses that we brought from Holland. I did not feel any discomfort from re-introducing dairy, such as strange gases, bloating or any other symptoms. My days off are definitely one of the positive things about these challenges, and today was a heavenly cheesy, milky, creamy day and I feel happy!

In retrospect

Once again, I really enjoyed editing the daily log entries and re-living these first 30 dairy free days. It was an extremely difficult month for me, and I have no doubt that I compensated for the lack of dairy with junky foods. Also, in retrospect, I realize that learning to eat in different ways takes time. Considering the importance and relevance of dairy in my diet normally, this was a significant month. I am sure that I learnt a lot this month about cooking without dairy or how to make the right snack choices. As important as dairy was, and is, in my diet, the truth is that this was the first month of a total of five dairy free months over a one year period. After completing the other four still upcoming consecutive dairy free challenges (dairy and gluten free, macrobiotic, paleolithic diet and vegan), I got so used to not having dairy that it didn't even cross my mind as a food choice. Today, almost two weeks after the challenges are over, I eat dairy on a regular basis, especially Greek yogurt with nuts and fruits, stinky and highly fermented cheeses, and butter in my recipes.

CHAPTER 6 – ALCOHOL FREE

I realized at some point in the last month that I have been able to drink alcohol throughout all my challenges so far. In fact, alcohol has often turned out to be the "go to" option at social gatherings, when my limitations did not allow me to eat most or any of what was being served. It is gluten free, coffee free, vegetarian, good beer and wine are whole foods, and it has no dairy. So now I feel that I can only gain from going one month without alcohol. To be honest, I don't think this will be too difficult. More importantly, after five months of food limitations, I feel the need to have a month that I can eat anything before number moving on to the seventh challenge. Especially because I already know what I want to do for month seven, and it is going to be extreme and tough. But I want to try it, even if it is the last challenge I do in this project. But first, let's see how alcohol free goes.

Day 1
I decided to start this challenge with a mini liquid detox, and therefore to eat only fruit and vegetables in liquid form for 36 hours. This means that for the time period starting last night before going to bed on night one, the entire day today, and a second night tonight, I can only eat fruit and vegetable smoothies and creamed vegetable soups. Although the beginning of the day went well, by late

afternoon I felt very tired and lacking in energy at now at night-time I have a bit of a dull headache at the back of my head. These symptoms may or may not be related to lack of calories. Regarding the alcohol free challenge itself, I did feel like an ice-cold beer in the afternoon while walking on the beach with my man, but nothing too difficult to overcome.

Day 2

I weighed in this morning and lost 0.5 kg in one day with my mini-detox. After eating a huge plate of oatmeal with nuts and raisins for breakfast, I got back my full energy levels, and already worked out, went for a long walk, and am right now actively working. But, I still can't get rid of the nagging headache at the back of my head.

Day 3

After feeling decently well in the morning yesterday, I spent the entire rest of the day nursing a wicked headache, as well as feeling nauseous and with an upset stomach. Must have gone for a dump (not diarrhea) about ten times in the last 24 hours and lost another 300 grams even though I have been eating normally. Not sure if it was the 36-hour detox, the re-introduction of dairy, or a virus. Today I have a bit of a stuffy nose, so it could very well be a virus. I did go to practice last night and felt ok energy-wise running around on the sand.

Day 6

Boy, I have never been as close to cheating in these challenges as I was this last weekend. It was very tough indeed! The reason being that we had a close friend, who lives in the UK and enjoys good wine and cold beer, staying with us for a few nights. Boy, it was oh-so-tough to watch him and Patrick enjoy great red wines while catching up while I sipped some herbal infusion. On top of that, we also had the last day of the National Ultimate beach ultimate league in which my team played 4 easily won games with a bunch of great beer drinking players. Man oh man… during the closing ceremonies, I actually felt pain in my chest and abdomen just thinking how good a cold beer would taste. I hung in there, but barely!

Day 13

Although I often get desires for a cold beer, a cold glass of white wine, or a gin and tonic, on a day to day basis this challenge is reasonably easy compared to the other ones. That being said, it is kind of funny how close I have been to cheating the few times that I am in a social situation in which everyone around me is drinking. The social aspect of drinking also has made me realize how difficult it must be for those who can't consume alcohol. For example, I went to the theatre with girlfriends from my book-club and felt a bit like a fundamentalist drinking sparkling water while everyone else was drinking wine during the break.

Day 18

Another very difficult weekend without falling off the wagon. I am actually curious about where that phrase comes from and am going to google it now, back in a second. Ok, found something that quenches my curiosity. According to google, the saying "falling off the wagon" supposedly originated in the late 19th century during the time of the Prohibition and refers to falling off the water wagon and therefore drinking alcoholic beverages instead of water (see, https://english.stackexchange.com/questions/37132/origin-of-the-idiom-falling-off-the-wagon). Funny that it actually makes more sense than I thought, since I always imagined that you needed to be drunk to fall off the wagon, making the saying nonsensical to me.

Anyway, this last weekend was again a true test in discipline and will power, and I repeat, it was hard not to fall off the water wagon. First, we had my niece's birthday party on Saturday night. Approximately 70 semi-intoxicated teenagers and a load of tasty and happy drinks… but not for me. And that is not all, this one was a double whammy! The day after the party, I played at the first women's beach ultimate tournament in Portugal on Sunday. AAARGHHHH…. I suffered a lot! One of the players who has been in Portugal for a few years and is going back to Germany, brought some great German beers to the field to cheer with the ladies. Oh man… I could only look, cheer the ladies with my water, and try not to weep from a self-imposed safe distance. I hate not being able to do what I feel like! AAARRGGHHH!!!!

Day 21

Today, I am starting to believe that this alcohol-free challenge is having a positive effect on me. I am extremely clear headed and strong and happy not to have cheated, not only in this current challenge but also for the last six months. Interestingly, I am also getting used to not drinking where I normally loved to do so. For example, last week at the book-club dinner with the ladies, where I usually drink copious amounts of wine, it was strangely and unexpectedly easy to stay wine-free. Hurray for that! Now, I am beginning to fear the next challenge, where the food limitations will be again a part of my daily life.

Day 25

The alcohol free 30 days are almost at an end and I am still not sure if I will have the capacity to do the diet regime that I planned to do next. I think I may be getting cold feet about what is to come. But one thing is for sure, I am really enjoying how I feel and how these challenges are empowering me to explore different foods and drinks.

Day 30

Here is the day, the last alcohol-free day! To be honest, I am more worried about if and how I will be able to do what I wanted to do as the seventh challenge than I am looking forward to having a drink.

Conclusion

On a day to day basis, being alcohol free was by far the easiest challenge of all the challenges so far. With that in mind, it was also the challenge that I came closest to cheating, particularly in three or four social situations where I just felt I "needed" a drink. I decided to take the almost physical pain I felt because I couldn't drink as a sign, and have therefore decided to decrease the amount of alcohol I ingest. Considering that I don't drink daily, this means less booze on party nights. Also interesting, I got used to and started enjoying having a clear head, especially at social get togethers when everyone around proceeded to get fuzzy. I am now curious to see how my alcohol consumption will change on a long-term perspective. Regarding my weight, I lost 0.6 kg this month (59.6 kg) as well as decreased 3 cm in waist circumference (83 cm). Not sure if the weight loss is completely alcohol related, as I am slowly getting back to my before-quitting-smoking weight of almost three years ago. Also, I find that I make healthier food choices and hand myself over to cravings less often if I have no restrictions. The waist circumference, however, is most likely at least partially alcohol related. Funny enough, today is my day off and I probably will not drink any alcohol. Actually curious to see how I will feel when I do…

Positives

- Again, I did not cheat even though I had a few close moments.
- Loved the fact that I could eat anything I felt like eating, especially after some months of food limitations.
- After overcoming moments of frustration, I started to enjoy feeling clear headed as everyone around me got fuzzy at parties.
- Found that great meals are just as nice with sparkling water and lemon.
- Enjoyed trying different homemade fruit and spice water infusions.
- Lost some weight and 3 cm waist circumference.

Negatives
- At parties and social gatherings, I often felt like a teetotaler (which means someone who abstains, or advocates abstaining, from alcohol - it is worth reading the origins of this word, try looking it up on Wikipedia).
- Missed out on tasting some excellent wines.
- Missed my occasional sunset drinks with my husband at the beach (although herbal tea was nice too).

My day off
Funny enough, I didn't drink any alcohol on my day off. Feeling powerful and clear headed and not necessarily needing or wanting a drink. Next challenge will allow me to have one single glass of white wine once or twice a week, but that will be it as far as drinks go for a while!

In retrospect
One thing is for sure, over the food-challenges year I seem to have lost the capacity to drink the way I used to. I still love my gin and tonics, good wines and cold beers, but one or two drinks and I am floating nicely... and quickly start feeling unpleasantly tipsy if I drink too much. This change is likely due to a bunch of factors, including weight loss, healthy eating, and, I would say mostly because of generally drinking a lot less and therefore lack of drink training. This alcohol-free month was not the first time going dry over the last few years. Before the world beach ultimate championships in Dubai in 2015, I did not touch alcohol or recreational drugs for 5 months. Also interesting is the reaction that I had after the 36-hour detox, including an upset stomach and headache, which is reminiscent to the first days of my intermittent fasting challenge in month 12.

H. Sofia de Campos Pereira

CHAPTER 7 – KETOGENIC DIET

After half a year of self-imposed food limitations, I feel ready as well as slightly anxious to start the seventh consecutive 30-day challenge, the ketogenic diet. There are a bunch of reasons I chose to do this regime at this time, but before I get into that let me describe the ketogenic diet and what it entails. I have been somewhat afraid of this diet, as it is, by far, the most radical of all the challenges I have done. The whole concept behind the ketogenic diet is that a diet high in fat and low in carbs as well as low in protein results in the body adapting to utilize fat instead of glucose for energy, through a process called ketosis. This diet has been used for over a century to manage seizures in patients with epilepsy, and sometimes works to control epileptic episodes in those who do not respond to pharmacological approaches. Considering the shift that the body and brain must undergo to use fat instead of glucose for energy, the ketogenic diet has a strong impact on the body as well as the brain. Lately, this diet has gotten a lot of attention from sports aficionados and athletes as a tool to re-shape the body, augment lean body mass (lose body fat), and influence endurance.

Before we get into how to eat on the ketogenic diet, I must bore you a little with the biology. Hang in there, and if you are truly not interested in the "why and how" of the crazy month to come, then feel free to skip the next two paragraphs. Here we go. The whole concept of fat adaptation is based on the fact that although our bodies and brains preferentially use carbs for energy, we have a much more limited amount of stored carbohydrate in our bodies than we do stored fat. The absolute maximum amount of carbs that our bodies can store (mostly in the form of glycogen stored in muscles and the liver) is 15 g per kg of body weight, with the average being closer to 500 g of stored carbs per person. This, at 4 calories per gram, translates into 2000 calories of stored carbs. Compare that to anywhere between 7-30 % of our body mass of fat (or more for so many overweight people) stored in the form of triglycerides. At 9 calories per gram of fat, this means that a very lean 60 kg person with 10 % body fat has 54 000 calories of stored fat in their body.

The much larger amount of energy available from stored fat taken together with the adaptive capacity of our body to use fat for energy supposedly results in a significant increase in long-term energy levels. In truth, our bodies often use fat for energy, such as in the morning after a low-carb meat and salad dinner, or when we fast for approximately 24 hours (or less if we are physically active).

In today's much publicized diets and lifestyles, there is a tendency to label very low carb diets as ketogenic diets. However, in a strict ketogenic diet, protein content must also be strictly controlled, as protein is quickly converted into glucose for our body to use for energy. For this month, I opted to go on a strict ketogenic diet, following the guidelines often administered to epileptic patients. This means that I will be ingesting less than 50 g of carbs a day (in the form of "over the ground" vegetables and some fruits), 1 g of protein per kg of body weight (in my case approximately 60 g of protein per day), and the rest of my daily calories in fat. If we do the math for a 2000 calorie a day diet, this means that I eat less than 200 calories in carbs, 240 calories in protein, and approximately 1600 calories in fat per day. Converting fat calories to grams, at 9 calories per gram, means 178 g of fat per day. That translates into a decent block of fat a day, more than one third of a pound!

To be honest, just the thought of eating this much fat without some starch to soak it up or protein to dilute it is making me slightly nauseous. Anyway, in the end, I am consciously choosing to go through with this. You may, as I have often done myself, question me as to why I am doing this particular challenge. I am not sure why, but perhaps because it is so different from my high grain diet. Or and also, perhaps because I am curious as to how the metabolic changes will impact my energy levels and/or thinking speed. Finally, I hope it will help me to lose a couple of kilos that have accumulated around my waist in the last few years. I have to admit, I am not looking forward to eating so much fat for a month, although I am curious to see how it goes.

Day 3

Three days of this new challenge have gone by and I am surprised that I still haven't had an alcoholic drink. Regarding the ketogenic diet itself, after a few days of eating loads of stinky high fat cheese, avocados, eggs cooked in butter, meat and cream, I am starting to think that this may not have been the wisest choice. Although I find it very interesting that I am not hungry at all. Quite the contrary, I feel constantly full and slightly nauseous. This is probably due to the specifics of fat digestion, which is very different to how we digest carbs or proteins and is generally a more prolonged process. Also, I am very surprised at how regular my intestines are… which is a good thing! Now going off to the market to buy some high fat stuff to cook, wish me luck!

Day 5

This entry marks the historical day where Donald Trump was elected the president of the United States. Oh my… I slept like crap because Patrick kept waking me up telling me Trump was ahead. When I did come upstairs in the morning, Tomas, our son, told me that he woke up at sunrise to his dad yelling at the TV while the final results were being announced. I went for a walk with my mom, but I can't seem to accept that this actually happened, I feel like the world has had a lobotomy. Hopefully writing here will distract me from this insane political and societal cluster f**k and get my energies and mind onto the things that I can control, namely food.

The truth is that after five days of eating a lot of fat and very little carbs (and limited protein) I am starting to feel a difference in my metabolism. Thankfully, the initial sick feeling I used to get just by thinking about eating fats is gone and I am surprisingly able to enjoy fatty meal after fatty meal. Thank goodness I am highly creative in the kitchen. Today I made pancakes with eggs and homemade walnut flour for breakfast and ate them with black berries. They were very good. For lunch, I had a green salad full of shrimp and mayo which also tasted great. All in all, I am never hungry and have a load of mental energy. Also, my intestines are working great. So, right now, all is good. Whereas a couple of days ago I thought I would never be able to do this diet for the entire month, at this point I feel confident that I will. I must be careful about what I choose to do in the 30 days afterwards to make sure I don't shock my system too much.

Day 11

After a positive period feeling great on the ketogenic diet (keto), I am once again just hanging in there. This is quite the radical diet and is not easy to follow at all. Amazing that after almost two weeks eating fat, I am still enjoying my fatty meals. The last days have been mediocre, I have been getting highly creative in the kitchen so that I can continue to enjoy eating the limited amounts of foods that I can eat. Lots of cheese, eggs, fatty meats, fatty fishes, nuts (some nuts, such as high carb pistachios and cashews are out), high fat yogurt, avocados, and greens. Although I don't believe in frequently weighing myself, this diet has just gotten me so curious that I had to weigh in, and found that I have lost 1 kg in 11 days. Considering that I am not hungry at all, exercising very little and eating a load of fat, I am shocked.

Regarding exercise, at this point I have an overwhelming lack of general energy and get somewhat nauseous when I try to push myself. I also notice that I am much lazier than usual after dark. There has been a serious stomach flu going around, which both my son and husband fell victims to, so that may explain some of the "keto flu" symptoms that have turned me into a couch potato the last few nights. Besides actively walking around during the day and a few bouts of intense 15 minute workouts, I have been very sluggish and have done very little. Tonight, I am going to play disc on the beach and am curious as to how I will feel.

Day 12

I didn't make it to practice last night because I felt that my muscles were extremely tired and weak… to the point that it was almost painful. Partially due to the physical lethargy I am feeling and partially due to my science mind, I decided to review the scientific literature discussing the effects of the ketogenic diet on athletic performance and brain function (see reviews and references at the end of this chapter). This post may therefore be a bit of a science lesson. If you are not interested in the fatty science, again, I apologize and suggest you skip this entry completely. If you are interested, and I hope that you are, then read on… I will try to make it worth your time.

From what I have found after much browsing and researching, there is no doubt that the ketogenic diet influences body composition and results in weight loss. On the other hand, there does not appear to be any advantages regarding athletic performance for athletes which are adapted to metabolizing fat after a period of adaptation on a ketogenic diet. The physical adaptive requirements and responses that influence athletic performance vary greatly depending on the type of sport, as you can see by the obvious differences between the body of an elite marathon runner compared to that of a wrestler or a heavy weight lifter. Regarding the effects of a ketogenic diet on long-term aerobic endurance, such as that required for marathon running, there seems to be no significant effects (some publications show slightly positive, some slightly negative and others no effects). Conversely, the majority of studies show that the ketogenic diet imposes negative effects on anaerobic "explosive" performance, mostly attributed to decreased glycogen storage in muscles and therefore limited capacity for anaerobic muscle contraction.

These results help make sense of how my body feels as well as are in accordance with my current knowledge and what I have read over the last few days. There is also the factor of the "perceived effort" by the athlete, which plays a significant role in athletic performance and seems to be negatively augmented by lack of available carbohydrates. If you are interested in food and athletic performance and would like to read further, I suggest taking a look at a Joint Position recently published by the Dietitians of Canada and the American College of Sports Medicine. Their comprehensive review of the literature clearly indicates that what is best for athletic performance is a whole foods diet rich in vitamins, minerals and nutrients. Furthermore, they also show which nutrition adjustments are most effective just before, during and after intense training or competition for various forms physical demands as well as numerous times of exertion.

Contrary to the effects, or lack of effects, of the ketogenic diet on athletic performance, there is strong evidence of the positive effects of this diet on other physical parameters. including neuroprotective effects on patients with Parkinson's, Alzheimer, or those that have suffered brain injury. Furthermore, when applied for a limited time, the classical ketogenic diet has positive effects on not alcoholic fatty liver disease and on reducing the levels of triglycerides in the blood. This brings me to an interesting point, I am shocked at how many people think eating fat is what causes high blood fat and high cholesterol, including many health professionals. It is currently known that the fat in our blood is mostly attributable to fat produced by our livers rather than ingested fat, and a significant proportion of the fat that our livers make comes from excess carbs that are not burned up by our body's energetic needs. Because so many people have been telling me that my cholesterol is going be crazy high due to my eating so much fat, I have decided get my blood lipid profile (cholesterol test) done at the end of this challenge.

Day 13

Almost at the end of the second week on the ketogenic diet and I continue to feel very tired, especially at the end of the day. In fact, I feel muscle fatigue to the point of a constant dull pain in my legs. Taken together with what I read about the ketogenic diet causing mineral imbalances due to loss of body water (hypo-magnesium, calcium, potassium, and sodium), I bought some multi-vitamins and minerals and started taking them today. Later this afternoon, I will do a work out and then later go to disc practice.

Day 14

Today, I am finally feeling a little bit better. What a relief, maybe I am finally getting keto-adapted. I do, however, have a headache, which I am not sure is related to this diet regime. It could simply be because I have my period, the atmospheric pressure (I am sensitive to this and it is a dreary grey day) or a virus. Yesterday, I was an absolute mess! I cancelled going to disc practice at the last minute because even simple walking tired me out. Normally on Thursdays I do volunteer work at the community center about a mile from home, and enjoy exploring different paths when walking back home. This was not the case yesterday, when the journey home felt impossibly long and I felt like an old and haggard lady as I dragged my feet all the way home. Worse than that, I kept fretting about how long it was taking to get to the next viewed milestone such as the pedestrian bridge I can see from some distance. The whole walk, which is usually a pleasure, was a serious chore. To add to that, I was edgy and impatient all day. I seriously considered cutting this experiment short. Thanks to a lot of encouragement and support from Patrick and my accountability coach, I am glad I hung in there.

Day 15

I decided to stop taking the vitamin and mineral supplementation, since they did not seem to help after taking them for two days. The lack of energy and lack desire to move mean that although I have been actively doing basic maintenance activities around the house (grocery shopping, walking to do chores, cleaning up the house, etcetera), I have not done any serious exercise this week. In fact, I have done very little physical activity this entire challenge.

On another note, I read an interesting fact about this diet regarding weight loss which I think is important to share with those choosing to do this to lose weight. It does require me to get a little into biology, I hope you are getting used to it. Recall the earlier discussion about carbs stored in the body in the form of glycogen? Well, this stored glycogen, which is typically close to 500 g in an adult, is associated with water at a 1:2 or 1:3 ratio in our muscles and our liver. As glycogen stores get depleted after some time without eating carbs, there is quick initial weight loss due to the glycogen being used up and the water associated with the glycogen lost. This means that up to 1.5 kg of weight loss in the first week is not due to fat burning but rather to glycogen and associated water being depleted. No wonder I feel like a raisin and look like crap! It will be interesting to see how the rest of the month goes and how quickly my weight resumes back to normal afterwards.

Day 17

Still hanging in there. Once again, getting creative in the kitchen so that I am not eating the same thing all the time. Made a "dessert" consisting of full fat cream, a quarter of a pomegranate and some plain bone gelatin. Tasted great with some high fat walnuts. Also, I went to the butcher and bought a large bone to boil up with some veggies to make a nice salty high mineral broth. Although I am still weak, I am starting to feel a lot better. After so many failed attempts, today I may I have the strength to work out, finally! Let's see how it goes.

Day 18

Last night, I did a short, 3-part intense exercise routine (thanks to

David and Filipa) which includes burpees, push-ups, V-ups and squats, and felt almost normal. Also, as far as cooking and eating goes, I am starting to adventure more with unsweetened coconut to get away from the fatty dairy. Still 12 days to go, but I think I will be able to stick with it. Tonight I will most likely go to play disc after some weeks off, and I am curious as to how I will feel running on the sand.

Day 19

Getting a bit more used to the diet and feeling less tired at the end of the day. Disc was cancelled last night, so I still haven't played or practiced since being on a ketogenic diet. I do feel strange sometimes, a bit dizzy and nauseous. Not enjoying this one.

Day 24

After three and a half weeks eating tons of fat, I am finally feeling my energetic self again! This is a good change from this last weekend, when I was again seriously thinking of giving up this crazy diet. I felt weak, unmotivated, sick of eating fat and was badly craving carbs, especially healthy whole grain carbs. And again, with the help of great friends, I managed to get over the hump. First, we had dinner with Moi and Inês, who is an amazing cook and prepared the most incredible ketogenic dinner, consisting of a slow roasting pork shoulder and lots of fantastic fatty chesses. Heavenly! Also, at Patrick's suggestion, I have decided to add a new challenge "within a challenge" to this last week - I will work out hard every day to test how I feel and to see if it makes an impact on losing accumulated body fat. Yesterday, I finally went to play disc. Although I felt quite dizzy at times and had to stop for a few moments, I could run on the sand and catch. Throwing was tougher as my arms felt weak and my balance a bit out of whack. The good news is that I feel committed and strong in my resolution to end this with a bang. Later on today, I will do a powerful weights and cardio routine at home. My weight has maintained at 1 kg less than when I started this challenge.

Day 29

I have had it with this diet, and want to quit now! Amazing that there is only one more day to go and I am nevertheless struggling to hang in there. Since today is Friday, I decided to get my blood work done this morning on an empty stomach. What an adventure that turned out to be! Right after waking up, I walked over to the local pharmacy on an empty stomach after an overnight fast for the blood tests. The result for my total blood cholesterol was 290 mg/dL, which is a little high, but within my normal parameters. However, the result for the blood triglycerides levels of 375 mg/dL was ridiculously high… butter in my veins! I came home quite unhappy at this unexpected result, especially after spending an entire month insisting that as unhealthy as this diet was, it was not going to raise my blood lipids. While eating my ketogenic breakfast of full fat Greek yogurt and walnuts, and frantically opening and reading up on more science, I decided that my triglyceride results were impossible. Especially considering that I typically have low triglyceride concentrations in my blood. Furiously, off I ran back to the pharmacy, now on a full stomach, and asked the pharmacist to repeat the test. She told me that since I had just eaten, my results would only be higher, and that my triglyceride results were not surprising since I had been eating fat for a month. So I made a deal with her, if the results of the second test were worse or the same, I would pay for the test again. However, if not, then she would refund my original 6 Euros. She agreed, and the second test resulted in a triglyceride measure of 199 mg/dL! Almost half of the initial test, and now with food in my belly and triglycerides quickly on the way from my digestive tract into my blood. Urghhh!

I did get my money back, but the whole experience was quite unsettling for me. Especially because it obviously indicated that the results of the blood work were inconsistent and therefore meant absolutely nothing! After bitching to Patrick about the whole thing, he suggested that I go to an accredited medical clinic and get the whole blood work properly re-done, even if the results were going to be altered by the fact that I had eaten within an hour of blood collection. Off I ran to the analysis clinic to insist with the nurse to take my blood quickly to avoid artefacts in the results. The nurse tried to talk me out of paying for the test, as my values would be off due to having eaten and would mean nothing. In the end, I won, and the results I got were mostly comparable to my normal levels from previous analysis. These were 290 mg/dL in total cholesterol (compared to 254 in 2015), 92 mg/dL in HDL (compared to 85), 174 mg/dL LDL (compared to 150) and 120 mg/dL triglycerides (compared to 84). And this, about one hour after eating a high fat meal, which may justify the slight increase in the level of my triglycerides, and in turn, total blood cholesterol.

Day 30
Last day, thank goodness! Hanging in there and not eating much today. Looking forward to a large bowl of oatmeal tomorrow!

Conclusion
This was, by a long shot, the most difficult and radical of all the food challenges so far, and the one that I needed the most support to not call it quits. For this, I must thank Patrick (my husband) for pushing me to start pushing my body physically even though I felt so tired, as well as my Health Coach, Patricia, for supporting me and incentivizing me to stick with it. I learnt a lot this month about foods and diets. Also, I read a load of science on ketosis and the effects of this diet. In the end, although it was very difficult, I now consider that 2-4 weeks on a ketogenic diet to be a true detox (I like the term ketox). The reason I say this is because when in ketosis, the body is forced to utilize and therefore renew fat stores, something that rarely happens when there are carbs available to meet bodily energy needs. Also, there is something about a keto adapted brain, or a brain getting its energy to function from fat. As bad as my body has felt, my brain has been sharp and on.

This has not been a great month as far as exercise is concerned. Excluding the last week, where I pushed myself to work out and to play disc, I didn't do much physical activity and felt weak and tired. Regarding weight loss and waist circumference, I lost 2 kg between the first and last day of the diet (weighing in at 57.6 kg) and 1 cm waist circumference (82 cm). Keep in mind, this weight loss can at least partially be attributed to loss of water from my body. In fact, I have felt dry and dehydrated many times this month, no matter how much water I drank or salt I ate.

Positives

- What a learning experience this month was! I often felt that I was my own lab rat and part of a crazy experiment. In the end, I am proud to have stuck with it.
- I got highly creative shopping for and cooking with high fat foods, and made fun recipes and soups that were enjoyable even when the whole idea of eating fat made me nauseous.
- I slept great throughout the entire month and maintained regular bowel movements.
- It was very interesting to feel the physical effects of ketogenic adaptation. For me, it took about three weeks to feel normal and somewhat physically powerful.
- My brain function seemed to improve. I felt very sharp, quick thinking and creative.
- Lost some weight, although at least 1 kg is only water.
- Detoxed. After this month, I believe this diet to be highly anti-inflammatory and a good shock to the system when done at the right time and in the right way. It is likely that I will use it periodically on myself throughout my life.

Negatives

- For the first three weeks, I felt very weak and had no physical energy for exercise.
- I felt nauseous many times, and got sick of eating fat.

- Although there were always options of something to eat, this diet is oftentimes very limiting and often unpalatable.
- I found this diet extremely difficult to do and maintain.

My day off
I am oh-so-glad to be eating normally again. Happily, I don't feel at all like junk food. Relishing in whole grains, fruits, and sweet potatoes.

Afternote (February 7th, 2017): A cousin who is also a close friend of mine suffers from "cluster headaches", and has episodes of nightly incapacitating headaches for periods of time that can last up to five months. In desperation and on my suggestion, he tried the ketogenic diet. Interestingly, after three days he started to notice changes typically associated with breaks in the cycles of headaches, such as variation in the time of day the headaches set in (in his case in the middle of the night to around dinner time) and alterations in their intensity. After one week, he finally had one pain-free night. Due to the difficulty in maintaining this diet long-term, he did not continue the ketogenic diet, but I thought this experience worth the mention.

In retrospect
The ketogenic challenge was not an easy chapter to edit. Although I could tell that my brain was on by the quality of my writing needing little adjustments, I am right now slightly nauseated just from reliving the experience. It was not easy an easy 30 days! On the other hand, it was a huge learning experience and probably the challenge that I learnt the most from out of the entire year. Looking back now, I think it was the month that had the biggest impact on my body and mind. It was also the challenge that inspired me to keep going on this food anthropological journey, since after being able to stick to this way of eating for 30 days I felt that I could take on any food challenge.
Regarding the long-term effects of eating 75 % of my caloric

intake from fat for 30 days, I now believe this experiment influenced my metabolism and that my body is currently better adapted to burning fat. I often eat "keto friendly" very low carb and high fat meals, especially as the first and/or last meals of the day or on days like today that I am mostly focused on the book and therefore doing very little physical activity. In sum, I will apply what I learnt this month throughout my life. It is unlikely that I will do a strict ketogenic diet as drastically or for as long as I did this month, but am now a full believer in the physical and mental health promoting properties of a periodic "ketox-detox" reset. Also, I am convinced that having undergone this experience helped me adjust quicker to the intermittent fasting 30-day challenge that I did on month twelve.

References

Dietitians of Canada: Nutrition and Athletic Performance: https://www.dietitians.ca/Dietitians-Views/Specific-Populations/Nutrition-and-Athletic-Performance.aspx

Gasior M, Rogawski MA, Hartman AL 2006. Neuroprotective and disease-modifying effects of the ketogenic diet. Behavioural Pharmacology, Vol. 17, pp. 431

Helge JW. 2002. Long-term fat diet adaptation effects on performance, training capacity, and fat utilization. Medicine and Science in Sports and Exercise, Vol. 34, pp. 1499

Rebecca CS, Crawford PA. 2012. Low-carbohydrate ketogenic diets, glucose homeostasis, and nonalcoholic fatty liver disease. Current Opinion in Clinical Nutrition and Metabolic Care, Vol. 15, pp. 374

Thomas DT, Erdman KA, Burke LM. 2016. Position of the Academy of Nutrition and Dietetics, Dietitians of Canada, and the American

College of Sports Medicine: Nutrition and Athletic Performance. Journal of the Academy of Nutrition and Dietetics, Vol. 116, pp. 501

H. Sofia de Campos Pereira

CHAPTER 8 – GLUTEN AND DAIRY FREE

Onto the eighth consecutive food challenge, no dairy and no gluten for 30 days! I am elated that the last challenge has come to an end and am almost giddy at the thought of eating carbs as a regular part of my diet again! After one month on the extremely hard to stick to ketogenic diet, I think this month will be a breeze. Funny how things change... how we change. In this case, my unexpected positive mind frame is a pleasant surprise, especially considering how difficult it was for me to do each of these two limitations separately in the not so distant past. Just to make sure that I keep track of weight changes for each challenge, I weighed myself this morning and weighed in at 58.6 kg. As expected, I gained back one of the two kilograms that I had lost last month, probably due to replenishing the carbohydrates on my day off, and therefore gaining back body storages of glycogen as well as the water associated with these stored carbs. This morning, my first bowl of oatmeal, made with vegetable milk, half a banana, rolled oats, seeds and cinnamon, tasted like heaven! After 24 hours of eating carbs, I feel completely different. My hair is shinier, my skin suppler, and my physical energy levels much higher. I am looking forward to this month, and to cutting out the cheeses and creams which I have been eating in excess for the last 30 days.

Day 3

As expected after a complete month on the ketogenic diet, I am finding gluten and dairy free easy and am loving eating whole grains and legumes again. I am in awe with the confrontation that the perception of difficulty when it comes to food limits, just like everything else in life, is relative. Theoretically knowing something is not the same thing as living it, and I am glad for this experience. Regarding how it feels to re-introduce carbs, I do have a slightly bloated stomach and a fair bit of gas, although I am eating very healthy whole foods. I had considered doing the paleolithic diet after the ketogenic, so as to re-introduce different macronutrients more gradually after a month of eating almost exclusively fat, but the thought of eating limited carbs for another entire month made me sad. So suffer I must, as my digestion tract and all its components need time to adjust. And that is ok.

Day 14

I can't believe two weeks have gone by without me having written about this food challenge. To be honest, although I have not cheated, it has not been easy to stay enthusiastic and faithful to no gluten and no dairy. After the strict ketogenic diet, the problem is not that I don't have enough choices of what to eat, because in comparison, I do have many choices. The problem is that I am starting to tire of the food limits and simply want to eat whatever I want to eat. This means that in order not to give up completely, I am back to frequently struggling with myself and fighting with my internal voices. When I am on the cusp of cheating, I start thinking to myself, "No one cares about your stupid food challenges," or "Why are you doing these dumb experiments?" It amazes me that it is the perception of how important or unimportant my actions are to others that come up as an excuse to cheat. On the other hand, the motivation to not cheat brings up a completely opposite inner talk, which is directed within and in the vein of "Hang in there, you can do it!" or "you have come this far, don't stop now". I wonder if there is a lesson to be learnt from this discrepancy between externally and internally oriented inner talks that can be applied to other parts of my life.

Regarding how I feel physically, the good news is that I feel great. I believe that I can get all the nutrients I need from the plethora of dairy and gluten free food choices. Furthermore, the consecutive and always changing food experiments have given me a huge amount of experience with different foods and cooking styles, so I feel completely happy spending time in the kitchen brewing up yummy dairy and gluten free stuff for me and the family to eat. I also think I look well. Healthy, full of energy and in a positive mindset. Now I just have to get through this momentary lull in will power and hang in there... oh, there it is again, I recognize that internally oriented positive motivation inner talk.

Day 21

Today is Christmas day, and since my mom is getting divorced and moving to a more sustainable apartment, it was the last family holiday celebration at the big house. I was afraid of the upcoming changes resulting in an overhanging negative or sad vibe, but there wasn't. We exchanged gifts, ate, drank wine, talked pleasantly, and were simply happy to be a family together. Regarding the food challenges, although it was tough not to eat all the yummy cream based deserts typical of a Portuguese Christmas meal, the turkey, rich nutty rice, and chestnut stuffing were great. And so, of course, was the wine!

Day 30

And here it is, the end of this challenge and very little to say. Unlike all previous challenges, this was less of a food challenge than an experiment in will power. Even though there were always options when it came to food, after eight months in this project, I am feeling saturated of the food limitations. New year was especially difficult. Patrick and I spent a few days in a very fancy hotel/spa in Algarve (Bela Vista, Portimão) where the most beautiful breads and cheeses were put out each morning for breakfast in a beautiful glass enclosed dining room surrounded by the ocean with its impressive rocky landscape. There were no gluten free starchy alternatives like oat or rice breads or crackers, so I had to satisfy myself with soft boiled eggs or eggs fried in olive oil and various wonderful types of fruit.

New Year's Eve dinner, which was celebrated with friends and their family, was also quite a challenge. Especially at desert time, where every amazing piece of cake or pudding was made with milk, cream and/or wheat flour. Although I still haven't done a month on the paleolithic diet (which I will hereafter interchangeably refer to as simply paleolithic or paleo), this challenge often felt similar to what paleo will be like. As such, I feel that I ate a lot of animal protein, vegetables and fruits this past month. Regarding my weight, I weighed in at 58.7 kg this morning, which is 100 g more that on the first day of this challenge. This is a good result, considering that we had Christmas and new year's holiday celebrations.

Conclusion

I don't have much to conclude about this month, and found that even if it was easy to do in regard to foods, it was a tough game of personal will power and strength not to give up and eat whatever I wanted. Unlike the last time I did gluten free for 30 days, beer was not an issue, and although I felt like a cold beer sometimes, it was easy to avoid. The thing I missed the most was cheese. I now realize how much I just love cheese. Today, on my day off, I immediately had some Dutch cheese accompanied by soft-boiled eggs for breakfast. In general, I found this challenge to be similar to a paleolithic style diet, especially when eating out of the house, and I am curious to compare it to my upcoming paleo challenge in a few months.

Positives

- It was very difficult to find "permitted" processed foods, due to wheat, dairy or both being in the ingredient list of most junk food.

- Found this challenge not difficult to do after the keto challenge, although this is probably true for any diet that follows a strict ketogenic diet.
- I felt energic and slept well.
- I feel very proud of myself for having managed to hang in there and stay with it through the seasonal festivities.
- Maintained my weight without dieting at all.
- Experimented with different foods, like for example making excellent oatmeal with nuts, banana and vegetable milks as well as an excellent black rice and seafood dish.

Negatives
- It was difficult to stay away from high quality cheeses and milky/creamy deserts, especially throughout the holidays.
- I believe that my body needs milk products to feel completely healthy, and am right now slightly fragile at the joints, although this may be because of age or because it's winter.
- I don't like limitations and am getting tired of not being able to eat whatever I feel like.

My day off
A dairy day from beginning to end. Cheese and eggs for breakfast, a Greek salad with Feta cheese for lunch, and a much-desired creamy pasta for dinner. Feeling good, and ready for one more dairy free month.

In retrospect
Before I get into how important I think this month was in terms of how it solidified the process that allowed for the completion of this project, I feel the need to mention that this challenge was followed by macrobiotic, paleo and vegan. This means that this was the first dairy free month of four in a row. After basically going four months without dairy, and looking back over my complaints of weakness in the joints during this month, I must clarify that these

did not persist and were therefore not due to lack of dairy. As I mentioned at some point in my entries during this experiment, I found this month to be more about gaining momentum to stay with the project than about the challenge itself. I am not sure where my brain was at this point regarding what I was expecting for the final outcome of these challenges to be. I don't remember if I had decided that I was going to write a book, but I think it was approximately during this time that the possibility of turning my logs into a book arose.

The book brings me back to the significance of the process that allowed for the eventual completion of this project. There are two friends (Pedro Vargas and Rui Pires) from my beach ultimate world that I consider gurus and with whom I love to discuss performance and sport psychology. They have been present, at least periodically, throughout the entire challenges year, and I have thoroughly enjoyed talking to them both. When I bounced the paragraph about inner talk and motivation with Pedro on messenger to see if it made sense, he replied – and resilience results from a balance between intrinsic and extrinsic motivation. This led to a whole conversation about the difference between being task (process) oriented or goal (outcome) oriented. Using sports as an example, and simplifying things, an outcome oriented athlete works to win, whereas a task oriented athlete works to improve a specific task or to better a previously obtained goal. For me, and using dairy free as an analogy, this was another task, or part of the process, that was successfully met. In the end, the eighth task of twelve which allowed me to reach the final goal of completing the year. This book, as the outcome, was probably only considered to be a possibility at some point after successfully getting through this month. And this, was undoubtedly due to a lot of intrinsic (me) and extrinsic (my family and friends) motivation and support.

CHAPTER 9 - MACROBIOTIC

The ninth month of food experiments is going to be macrobiotic for 30 days. There are many reasons that I chose to do this challenge, including that it used to be the food and lifestyle mode of the founder of the Institute for Integrative Nutrition, Joshua Rosenthal, who through the coaching program has greatly inspired me over the last few years to explore my own food self. More great reasons are that macrobiotic is highly flexible in what I can eat. Moreover, it is a diet rich in whole grains, which I miss terribly after a keto month followed by a gluten free month. The origins of the macrobiotic diet are based on the ancient Japanese theory of yin and yang, with the general concept being that we should eat whole foods grown as locally and as organically as possible.

According to macrobiotic guidelines, whole grains make up most of what we should be eating (the base of the macrobiotic pyramid) and these should be complemented by plant foods such as beans, chickpeas, vegetables (excluding night shades such as tomatoes, peppers, asparagus, potatoes, eggplant and zucchini, which are to be avoided), fermented soybeans (such as soy sauce, tempeh, tofu, miso), some fruits (no tropical fruits), some seeds and nuts, seaweed and some fish. Red meat, chicken, dairy, coffee, alcohol, and eggs are to be avoided, as is any processed food. The only thing that I am worried about is the no dairy limit, as I feel it is an important part of my diet. This is exacerbated by the fact that I can see that dairy based foods are going to be scarce in the next three months, considering that I still want to try paleo and vegan after this month.

Day 1
Today I opened the computer and googled "Macrobiotic" as a search term. After opening the "Macrobiotic Diet" article on Wikipedia*, I was taken aback to read in the conceptual paragraph, "Macrobiotics takes a view of health which contradicts science (Clow B, 2001)". Thinking further about this statement and taking into account that the origin of macrobiotic dates back to 1797 Japan, this is actually not surprising. Not only has the way we eat greatly changed in the last two hundred years, there have been significant advances in our knowledge of nutrition and dietary science. Also, like many other "diet lifestyle/theories", the macrobiotic diet originated and initially developed in one geographical location. The health benefits of eating locally, or more specifically, plants that are growing around you, is a very valid point. However, it is just as important to realize that different things grow in different places around the world. I believe it is essential to consider cultural/geographical differences. For example, why should tropical fruits be avoided if you live in the tropics?

The one thing I find highly positive about this diet/lifestyle is that it is based on guidelines rather than absolutes. For instance, in the case of red meat, the macrobiotic approach would state that it should be avoided most of the time, rather than forbidding that red meat be eaten. Regardless of the merits and fails of this diet/lifestyle, there are some things that completely resonate with me and my philosophy surrounding food and the ritual of eating. I do think it is important to be grateful for each meal, as well believe in the benefits of chewing every bite carefully. Although 50 chews may be an exaggeration, we do eat too quickly. Slowing down, chewing properly, and enjoying our meals is important for our digestive and nervous systems. Anyway, so far, I am enjoying and looking forward to this experiment. I am also happy to be going to the Instituto Macrobiótico de Portugal (Portuguese Macrobiotic Institute) with my friend Noélia next Tuesday to learn more. On a fun note, today I made my first miso soup for lunch, with seaweed, bock choy and tofu. I loved it, although I did get complaints from the rest of the family that the house smelt like fish sauce. Also, I have already placed dried chickpeas in water to hydrate for cooking tomorrow.

Day 3

I feel like am gently rolling into the macrobiotic mind frame and am thoroughly enjoying the journey, which is reminiscent of a warm hug on a cold day. Lucky that I picked this time of year, the dead of winter, for this experiment. I am loving cooking as well as eating whole grains, softly cooked vegetables, legumes, and sometimes fish, slightly spiced with soy, salt, miso or seaweed. Also, I am enjoying learning about the cooking ware and cooking styles that should be taken into account in the macrobiotic diet. It has been great fun learning and using new cooking methods and ingredients. Yesterday I bought organic whole grain rice syrup. What a great natural sweetener, cheap and due to its lack of taste, very versatile!

Day 8

This week, I had the pleasure of going for lunch with a long-term scientist friend, Noélia, who knows a lot about macrobiotic and loosely follows a macrobiotic lifestyle. Our outing felt like a research fieldtrip, and I learnt a lot from her extensive macrobiotic training. We met and had lunch at the Portuguese Macrobiotic Institute, which is in a beautifully renovated old building in downtown Lisbon. I love the feel of the place; the food is always great and the environment is cozy and warm. They also have a small shop with books and food, so I bought some barley Miso and my friend offered me some seaweed and sesame salt to welcome me into this new experiment. In general, I am thoroughly enjoying this challenge and notice that it is triggering some significant changes in my food, cooking and eating. For one thing, I am chewing much more frequently per bite, which means that I eat much slower and am often the last one at the table with food on my plate. Also, I am in a very positive mind-frame even though I haven't been sleeping great the last week (too many monkeys making noise and playing around in my brain). I do feel that this is the perfect time for macrobiotic, not only because it is winter but also there are no frisbee tournaments or anything else that I need to be physically competitive for. In general, this diet makes me feel soft and warm and lovey. I do miss meat and cheese, but I know it's only for a relatively short time, so its ok.

Day 15

Half way through the macrobiotic challenge and I am now at the point that I miss eating meat, eggs, chicken, and milk products. Also, I find it frustrating to have to avoid sweet potatoes (yams), zucchinis, and avocados, which are normally a regular part of my diet. On a positive note, I do enjoy the whole grains and love to incorporate miso in my vegetable stews. Also, I like that there is some flexibility in macrobiotics for a little wine, beer, and some sweets such as softly baked apple crumble.

Day 25

I can't believe that there are only five days to go until the end of the ninth month of challenges. Although I am still enjoying this regime, I am very much looking forward to the next challenge, which will be almost the polar-opposite approach to eating – the paleolithic diet! But for now, off to cook more grains.

Day 30

Oh, I am happy that today is the end day and can't wait to bite into some eggs and meats. Also, I seriously plan to load up on dairy on my day off, since dairy has been off-limits the last two months and will continue to be so for the next few challenges. My husband Patrick went to Holland a couple of weeks ago and brought back some wonderful cheeses that are patiently waiting in the fridge for me. I guess that for the next few challenges days off will be dairy days!

Conclusion

What a wonderful experience this month was. I loved learning about macrobiotic, and mostly found the foods and lifestyle guidelines to be a very pleasant experience. Especially during these cold and rainy winter months. I do think that it helped that I was going through a non-physically demanding phase of the year, without any competitive events and without any demanding muscle stimulation/strength training, and so did not feel the need for meat protein too much. Also, I did enjoy fish on average twice a week. Interestingly, I found there to be some similarities and overlaps between Portuguese food and macrobiotic, especially the legume dishes such as bean stew and chick-pea dishes, as well the potted fish and rice dishes or vegetable stews.

Regarding my weight, I did lose 1.4 kg this month, weighing in at 57.3 kg this morning. This is less than at the end of the keto month although my waist circumference is the same as it was then, measuring in at 82 cm. Overall, although I enjoyed macrobiotic, I am getting tired of having food limitations of any kind. Nine months is a long time, enough time to make a human baby. On the other hand, somehow the limits have opened new paths, and I have learnt a load about cultures, foods, and myself in this process.

Positives
- Enjoyed incorporation macrobiotic spices into my cooking, especially miso, seaweed, and sea salted sesame seeds.
- Once again, it was a pleasure finding alternatives to satisfy my sweet tooth. One great new sweetener that we are all happy for the discovery of is rice jelly. It is affordable, and if I must eat something sweet, I like to vary the sources and use various dark sugars, honey, maple syrup, etcetera. After this month,

rice jelly will surely become a regular in my pantry. Very good indeed.

- Felt great energy, slept well and maintained regular intestinal health throughout the month.
- Lost a bit of weight without any effort, which may be due to muscle loss because of the lull in serious training lately... but I feel good and feel that I look good.
- I really enjoyed some of the macrobiotic inspired "behavioral adaptations" around food, such as consciously appreciating the meal at hand. And practicing mindful eating, including trying to chew 50 times per bite. Probably closer to 20 or 30 for me, but I did notice changes.
- Loved eating grains again, which I really missed after the last challenge and will likely miss terribly in the upcoming paleo month.
- Very interesting to see that although my diet was 60 % grains, I felt no pain.

Negatives
- As in previous dairy-free months, it was very difficult to stay away from high quality cheeses and yogurts. This is especially complicated for me because I believe milk products are an integral part of my diet. Dutch cheese and yogurt are still a part of our household and my family's diet, I just can't eat either. Unlike the previous month, my joints felt ok without dairy, perhaps because I have not been training intensively this month.
- Besides the fact that I don't like limitations, I found some of the theories of macrobiotic dubious at best. Mostly because its origin is that of a whole food diet in Japan in the late 1700s, and therefore it is not applicable to all places. For example, why could I not eat avocados or sweet potatoes when they grow just outside my house? Sometimes I found this diet to be a bit silly and not necessarily health promoting. But this, I

believe, is usually the case when any feeding limitation is imposed by what we hold as being the truth from preconceived notions. Food limitations should be based on respect for our bodies, exploring new foods, and learning how we react to certain foods.

My day off

Once again, I overdid it on dairy, especially knowing that there are another two "dairy free" challenges coming up. It felt great to eat whatever I wanted, especially cheese and meat!

In retrospect

Reading over this month, I had forgotten how much I enjoyed macrobiotic and the large influence this challenge had on the types of ingredients readily available in the house. It was very nice to have an old science friend, Noélia, to teach me about the basic concepts of this diet/lifestyle and to accompany me on a field trip to the Portuguese Macrobiotic Institute, a place that I very much like. That reminds me, I am going to invite my friend and accountability coach, Patricia, to go there for lunch in the next few weeks.

With all this talk about macrobiotic foods and since I hadn't had lunch yet, I was immediately inspired to make a "macrobiotic-fusion-style" hummus, with sesame, organic sea salt, barley miso, olive oil, softly roasted garlic, and chickpeas. I am enjoying it right now over a bed of salad and wondering why this month was so easy... drifted by... came and went without any major bumps, slumps, or moments of desperation. I guess that is why it didn't leave a strong impression on me. I'm glad I got the opportunity to edit and re-live it, as it brought a pleasant experience that had been archived somewhere in the attic of my brain to the fore-front of my mind.

References

From Wikipedia*: Clow B (2001). *Negotiating Disease: Power and Cancer Care, 1900-1950*. McGill-Queen's University Press. p. 63. Before we explore medical reactions to therapeutic innovations in this era, we must stop to consider the meaning of 'alternative medicine' in this context. Often scholars use the term to denote systems of healing that are philosophically as well as therapeutically distinct from regular medicine: homeopathy, reflexology, rolfing, macrobiotics, and spiritual healing, to name a few, embody interpretations of health, illness, and healing that are not only different from, but also at odds with conventional medical opinion.

*This reference was cited in a log entry dated January 5, 2017. The Wikipedia article for "Macrobiotic Diet" has since been altered and the conceptual basis no longer contains this reference nor the statement that the macrobiotic diet contradicts science. (June 28, 2017)

CHAPTER 10 – PALEOLITHIC DIET

The tenth challenge and the one that I have been most curious about is finally here, the paleolithic diet, hereafter also referred to as paleo! There is an image forever engraved in my mind's eye associated with the first time I heard of this diet, which was during the health coach training program at the Institute for Integrative Nutrition. The lecturer, a strong advocate of the paleo diet/lifestyle, was a testosterone empowered man dressed in a tight black t-shirt and jeans, with a faux-hawk and lots of muscles. Whilst walking around on stage like a caged large feline and talking about how we have lost our full potential as humans, he showed an image to make his point. This image, which did I mention I will never forget? was of a chihuahua dog and a wolf, and was used to show the transformation of our "full potential selves" (the wolf) into the modern-day man (the chihuahua dog) incurred by our actual-day eating habits. I loved the dramatic effect of his delivery, his male strength, and even some of the theory. Speaking of the theory, the paleolithic diet is very rich in theory, so please bear with me as I go into it before diving into my cave-woman experience. Again, skip it if you wish, although I really hope you don't.

The Paleolithic period extends from the earliest known use of stone tools by our ancestors, circa 2.6 million years ago, to approximately 10 000 before the present time. It was during the Paleolithic era that the anatomically and behaviorally "modern" human is believed to have emerged in eastern Africa circa 200 000 before the present time, having gradually evolved from early members of the genus *Homo* into modern and much larger brained humans (*Homo sapiens sapiens*). Regarding our dispersal, we started expanding throughout the planet by around 50 000 before present, initially making it to Europe and Australia, followed by Japan, Siberia and eventually to the Arctic Circle. By the end of the Paleolithic, humans had crossed from what is today modern Russia to modern Canada and quickly expanded throughout the Americas.

Nearly all of our knowledge of Paleolithic human culture and way of life comes from comparisons to modern tribal cultures who live as contemporary hunter-gatherers, similarly to their Paleolithic predecessors. As far as we know, humans grouped together in small societies consisting of less than 100 individuals, and subsisted by gathering plants, fishing, hunting or scavenging wild animals. One interesting aspect of the hunter-gatherer lifestyle that drastically changed in future Neolithic farming societies and modern industrial societies is that Paleolithic humans enjoyed an abundance of leisure time. As a small aside, I have to admit that I like this fact, although boredom has become a luxury in the digital age, I believe we need to be bored at times to be at our best. A little boredom is health promoting as well as allows for great creative thoughts. Especially in children, who will come up with the coolest things to do when bored. Bored comments aside, let's get back to paleo. My highly critical scientific mind has a tough time swallowing the concept of defining a diet/lifestyle based on a period of human history encompassing more than 2 million years as well as a geographical area covering most of our planet. Just think about how much has changed in how we eat over the last 150 years, or the cultural differences that exist between our food ingredients and cooking styles across continents today. And this in a global society, where information exchange can travel over large geographical regions in merely seconds. And, to add even more entropy to the paleo dietary concept, there were significant geographic and climatic changes during the Paleolithic era (Pleistocene epoch of geologic time) which had large effects on pre-human and human societies, obviously including on their food and feeding.

Paleo supports the paleo diet/lifestyle as ideal because they believe that not enough time has passed for our biological systems to have evolved to deal with foods products from agriculture, which started approximately 10 000 years ago. Therefore, according to the paleo theory, foods from crops such as grains and dairy from domesticated animals are highly detrimental to our health. What I find particularly interesting, and this is a small scientific aside that I can't resist telling you, is the comparatively recent evolution of the B antigen in human blood, which is present in people with blood types B or AB. The B blood antigen is believed to have initially appeared between 10,000 and 15 000 years ago in the Himalayan highlands. Since the B blood antigen has been estimated to have initially appeared at the time when farming started, it is often associated with dairy tolerance. Also, and continuing to refute strict paleo, there are other putative reasons for the significant increase in our brain size during the paleolithic era. For example, think about the increase in mobility and therefore augmented exposure to different environments, foods, shelters, social systems and so on that occurred when we came out of the trees. Like everything human, it is never simple.

Ok, now that some of the science as well as my doubts and criticisms of the theoretical basis behind this eating style are out of the way, let us go along with the premise that we can define a paleo "hunter and gatherer" diet. This diet should probably be considered a modern version of what was consumed when our brains went through their greatest expansion. That's what this month will be about, the "modern paleo" diet. Since I cannot eat foods from agriculture, that means that grains or sugars are off limits, although I would bet you that any caveman gorged on all the ripe fruit or honey combs that he/she came across. But I do believe that sugars are a drug, at least for most of the population, and that there would be much less inflammation and auto-immune disease in our population if they were used as such. Regarding what I am allowed to eat on the paleo diet, there is some controversy regarding consumption of dairy, and so I intend to follow a strict version of no dairy except for clarified butter that has no lactose and is highly similar to meat fat in nutritional content. Of course, processed foods are not allowed. I will therefore be eating organic meats and fish, nuts, all veggies (except potato), low glycemic index fruits, and eggs. Considering that I cannot eat grains or legumes, this diet is basically the polar opposite of macrobiotic.

As a diet/lifestyle, the paleo diet is very popular right now. I think I can safely venture to say that with paleo cook books, ingredients, courses, sports bars, etcetera, it is a multimillion dollar industry. Athletes love it as the high protein content in this diet is ideal for muscle synthesis and therefore aids in getting "pumped". Housewives love it because it is great for thinning out. Personally, I am looking forward to this month. To add incentive to this challenge, I have joined the gym and intend to hit the weight room hard with Melissa's Ultimate Athlete Project workouts. As a cavewoman at the gym, I hope to increase my lean body mass and shed a little more body fat, which will hopefully result in better explosive performance playing disc.

Day 1

One day into my cave-woman month and I am already missing grains and dairy. This is not going to be easy. On the other hand, I do get to eat all kinds of yummy things that I like (it's a good thing that I am an optimist). Speaking of good foods and cooking ideas, I went online to look for what I paleo foods that I may like to make and eat. While searching for recipes on Pinterest using "paleo" and "recipes" as search terms, the incredibly high number of search results flabbergasted me. Considering that it is supposedly a caveman diet, I also found it amusing to see that most of paleo recipes were highly elaborate and appetizing. Also very funny, there were loads of recipes for "paleo breads, cakes and muffins", which in itself is contradictory considering that baked goods were invented as a way to eat grains from crops (fermented grains). Anyway, I look at the amazing fancy images of paleo cooking and it makes me laugh to imagine caveman internet and fancy cooking apparatus like blenders, juicers and ovens. In a way it's good news for me, considering that raw meat and raw nuts are just not that appetizing.

Day 3

I have never eaten so much meat in my life, I almost feel like growling! Seriously, although I thoroughly enjoy meat, fish and nuts, this diet has too much animal protein for me. Also, even though I eat whenever I'm hungry, I miss the complex starchy carbs and legumes to the point that I often feel slightly unsatisfied. The one thing I have noticed is that this diet is very expensive. This is especially true because it is important for me to eat high quality meats and fish, which means that I only buy organic meats and wild salmon. Taken together with the nuts and berries, this is not a diet for the economically challenged.

Regarding fitness, I have joined a gym close by with Patrick and my daughter Sara. After my evaluation at the gym this week, I made a conscious decision to reduce my body fat and increase muscle mass. I really believe paleo will help. In a way, this eating regime reminds me of the ketogenic diet from a few months ago, although without the high fat dairy and allowing for a lot more fruits and vegetables. Although I do miss my grains and dairy, I am nowhere near to cheating.

Day 7

After one week as a cave woman and I am rocking paleo! Of course, nothing is mono-factorial, and I am sure that part of the reason I feel like I do is because I joined the gym and am regularly exercising in the weight room as well as playing or practicing disc at least twice a week.

Day 12

Besides the fact that it is extremely difficult not to dig my teeth into the freshly baked bread that is staring at me every morning at the local bakery, I am still enjoying paleo. In fact, much more than I thought I would. During the first week, I missed starches and often felt that although I was not necessarily hungry after a meal, something was missing. However, I have found ways around this by baking paleo friendly pancakes, tortillas, and even cakes made from bananas, eggs, coconut oil (or olive oil) and then various seeds and nuts pulverized (or not) into flour. Very good indeed! I am actually enjoying this so much, and feel so good, that I am starting to dread the idea of trying vegan next month. Hmmm, I am having a ha-ha moment, maybe I will go vegan-paleo… that will definitely get the extra fat off my stomach area.

Day 22

I am still thoroughly enjoying being a cave-woman. And even though it is not easy to stay away from starches or legumes, I feel great and powerful. Funny that I also think that this diet is influencing my behavior by specifically increasing my directness. In fact, sometimes I'm surprised about what comes out of my mouth and almost want to look back and see who just said that (me?). Also, I notice that this eating regime is affecting my entire family immensely. My husband, who is an avid meat lover, has been enjoying going out of his way to make great paleo meals. We also bought a small "veggie peeler" that can cut vegetables into spaghetti like strings, which is fantastic for making zucchini noodles (zoodles). I can't believe that there is only one more week to go and am not looking forward to the next and second-last challenge. But until then, I still have a beach ultimate tournament to play as a cave-woman. Curious to see how playing seven games over two days without any simple carbs between matches goes.

Day 30

Playing a tournament on a strict Paleo diet was not easy. I felt great going into the tournament, full of energy, strong and in shape. Considering my team was the organizational team and therefore had to set up fields, tents, and all other sorts of organizational activities as well as play, the weekend was very physically challenging. What I did find was that it was impossible for me to maintain the same amount of energy for four games in a row without eating some quick digestion starchy carbs. I didn't, but felt increasingly tired as the day went on. The night after the first day, and after a complete Paleo dinner of meats and fruits, I felt very sleepy and in need of something else to eat. But thank goodness, I got into the people and the party and continued on my dancing paleo way. By bedtime, I was thoroughly happy with the day and internally laughing while re-living the random moments that you often experience with the frisbee crowd. Luckily for me, the challenge ended on the first day of the tournament and the second day was my day off, which means that I could eat anything. And, better yet, drink beer with my team after the games were over.

Conclusion

I was surprised what a great month it was eating like a hunter and gatherer cave-woman. For one thing, I did not expect to enjoy eating so much animal protein, which was truly a pleasure! In a sense, I have to laugh when I think of the fancy amazing paleo recipes that both Patrick and I concocted this month, nothing "cavey" about these meals. Also, I do tend to eat slowly and chew a lot lately, also not an eating behavior I visualize as being how our ancestors ate. The modern paleo is all about adapting to the modern world, and this diet/lifestyle has adapted quite well to the western society's current need to cut down on pro-inflammatory foods. As I mentioned before and think is important to note, although the quality of foods that the paleo diet supports is excellent, with all its nuts and meats, this regime is not light on the wallet. Also, it is not a diet that is light on the planet. As far as the environmental footprint, our current meat industry places a heavy load on our environment. We should be eating more plants, and we should be able to take advantage of the great healthy gains that we can get from grains and legumes. Ha-ha, that is a great saying! Great gains from grains...Try to say that three times in a row without screwing up!

Regarding my physical self, I felt great during this paleo month. I had plenty of energy and strength for my active daily life, including training, working, and enjoying my family. Regarding the effects of the paleo diet on athletic capacity, in an interesting review of the merits of popular diets on weight loss and athletic performance, Rosenbloom (2014) states that although all weight-loss diets work in the short term, there do not appear to be long-term benefits of any of these, including paleo, on athletic performance. Furthermore, the author states the importance for athletes to recognize the limitations inherent to specific diets and work with a sports dietitian to modify feeding plans to meet their unique needs. In this vein, although I was strong and feeing fit all month at the gym and playing disc, the one exception was on the first day of the two-day beach ultimate tournament, where I really felt the need for quick digesting carbs. I did thin out a bit more this month, and now weigh in at 56.7 kg and have a waist circumference of 78 cm. That is a 600 g weight loss and a 4 cm loss in waist circumference. Of course, these results are likely influenced by the regularity of my physical activity, which include regular sessions of strength training at the gym (four times per week) and disc (at least two times per week).

Positives
  - Surprisingly, I thoroughly enjoyed eating so much meat, fish, and eggs.
  - As with all previous challenges, it was a pleasure to find alternatives for my sugar cravings and therefore to became an expert at making sweet potato pancakes and cookies.

- Just like with most of my challenges, I felt great energy, slept well and my intestines were amazingly regular. In fact, I did notice a difference in the quickness and regularity of bowel movements. Paleo power dumps!
- Felt fantastic at the gym and that my body responded well to physical strength and conditioning training. Also, and probably related, I lost 600 g and 4 cm waist circumference. In general, I feel like my body is getting where I want it to be... I feel increasingly good and feel that I look good.
- Very interesting to see that I can live without the products of agriculture. Considering how difficult my initial gluten free month was, I am pleasantly surprised at how much easier this month was, even though I could not eat rice or any other grain.
- It was very difficult to find unhealthy food choices with paleo.
- All in all, this challenge was an unexpected wonderful experience.

Negatives
- As with all the other challenges that exclude dairy foods, it was very difficult to stay away from high quality cheeses and yogurts. On the other hand, I must emphasize that even though I have been doing regular strength and disc training, I did not have pain in my joints without dairy.
- Also, and a recurring theme when it comes to food regimes, I found some of the theories behind paleo comical at best. Especially considering the fancy recipes that were served up to my family this month.
- Paleo is expensive.

My day off
Wow, I ate a load of cheese on my day off! And beer! It was wonderful to bite into the dry bits and corners of wonderful Dutch cheeses that had been waiting in the fridge for me to be out of the

paleo month. And beer, oh boy did beer taste good! Oh so good! I spent my whole day off playing beach ultimate at a tournament, organizing, drinking beer, and eating anything I felt like (bread with Nutella tasted awesome). Since it was the second and final day of the tournament, which is hosted by our team, we finished off the day at a restaurant celebrating. The tournament is called Lisbon MOW, and is fantastic thanks to the impressive and highly positive organization from two teammates, Carla and Dani, who are also great friends. Way to end my cave-woman month... eating pizza and cheesecake accompanied by sweet Lambrusco wine with the team. OMG, that was awesome!

In retrospect

Before I get into the highly positive aspects of the paleolithic diet, bear with me as I lay one more recent scientific finding on you that I immediately found relevant while reading it a couple of weeks ago. There is now evidence that we started using tools much earlier than previously thought, since ancient stone tools dating back to 3.3 million years, which is pre-paleolithic, were recently found in Kenya. This puts in question previously calculated chronological estimates of when our brains started expanding, which may have occurred earlier than we previously thought. Regardless of the flaws in the whole concept of being able to define a diet that encompasses over 2 million years and the entire planet, our modern concept of paleo was a pleasure to do. I was not expecting to enjoy this month half as much as I did. I felt great, loved the foods, and was completely surprised by Patrick's coming on board and loving being a cave-man too. At least at dinner time, when he made the most amazing and tasty meals, including the now family favored noodles from zucchini (zoodles).

Regarding our health, there are huge advantages to paleo, mostly because agriculture is banned and therefore processed foods are out. Did it have a long-term effect on the way we and I eat? Yes. Whether by itself or in combination with the ketogenic and gluten free challenges, it definitely did! I eat paleo meals often nowadays. Also, I no longer consider the need for starchy accompaniments such as bread, rice, potatoes, or pasta in my meals. For example, for dinner tonight, Patrick made a fantastic zoodle dish with shrimp and a lime-coconut creamy sauce for dinner. Another big change is that I eat eggs much more often than I used to, and eggs with many vegetables is a oftentimes a family breakfast or lunch favorite. Taken together, this means that there are noticeable differences in how long bread lasts in our household in comparison to what it used to last.

References

Rosenbloom C. 2014. Popular Diets and Athletes Premises, Promises, Pros, and Pitfalls of Diets and What Athletes Should Know About Diets and Sports Performance, Nutrition Today, Vol. 49, pp. 244

Wong K. 2017. The new origins of technology. Scientific American, Vol. 316, pp. 22

CHAPTER 11 – VEGAN

Here we are, on the second-last and much dreaded eleventh month of 30-day food challenges, no animal products. I never thought I would be able to go vegan, and to be honest, I am slightly reluctant... especially after enjoying being a cave woman for a month. On the other hand, I have gained a load of experience cooking and eating animal food alternatives this year and am looking forward to the challenge. There are many who strongly advocate the health benefits of a vegan diet, and if you are interested in learning more about this I would suggest reading the book The China Study by T. Colin Campbell and Thomas M. Campbell and/or taking a look at https://www.forksoverknives.com/.

There is no doubt that if we all consumed a vegetable based diet, our footprint on the planet would be much less damaging. Just think of the huge number of calories in plant material that is necessary to feed a cow. Also, our current animal rearing practices are mostly focused on high production rather than quality. If our meat was coming from animals that are grazing in the fields and therefore returning nutrients back into the ground through their feces that could then be used for crop plant fertilizer, that would be ok. But mostly, our meats come from animals which have been fed grain based feed, which is not their natural food, as well as have been reared on hormones and antibiotics. We also waste a lot of food product at many levels along the production and consumption chain from live animal to the store to the table and then our guts.

Regardless of the many merits of a vegan diet for our planet, this month represents the first of the twelve challenges that has some serious nutrient deficiency issues. First, it lacks vitamin B12, which we can only get and bio-assimilate from animal based foods. Considering that we can store vitamin B12 in our livers for years, I will try not to supplement for the next month. Also, I am slightly worried about the decrease in healthy fish fats that I will be eating (EPA and DHA Omega 3) and how that will affect my eyesight, especially at nightly practices on a somewhat lit beach. Of course, there is plenty of Omega 3 in plants, but not the longer carbon chained EPA and DHA, which I normally get a plenty of from my frequent sea food meals.

Day 1

Initiated my vegan month with a fantastic breakfast consisting of oatmeal made with almond milk and topped with loads of cinnamon, fruits, and nuts. Tasted great! I also started soaking some beans to make a rich bean soup. I am curious about how much I will miss meats and fish and am going to try not to eat too much grains this month. Today, I am still physically exhausted from the tournament, but tomorrow I hope to hit the gym and see how I feel.

Day 2

Only two days have gone by and I am already hating the limitations imposed by this regime, especially when eating out. Yesterday was a friend's birthday and all I could eat at her party was chips and breadsticks, having to forego wonderful octopus and shrimp dishes as well as a fresh mushroom quiche and amazing cheeses. Today I feel bloated and low in energy. On the positive side, I went shopping this morning for fresh greens and filled up a large bag with wonderful food for merely 7 Euros. This would be an impossible feat on the paleo diet.

Day 4

Feeling slightly gassy and bloated on day four as a vegan forager. Over the past two days, I have been eating a lot of healthy greens and legumes and avoiding breads and flour in general. I think my microbiome is going through a roller coaster ride and may take a while to adjust to the radical change in diet. Let's see how I feel in two weeks. This month, there are a lot of close friend and family birthday celebrations, which can be socially difficult as a vegan. Yesterday, I took a friend's suggestion and ate dinner at home before going to a family dinner party (thanks Chris!). It was an interesting social experience to hang out at the party, enjoying chatting and eating salad. Funny that no one noticed that there was anything different or odd about my eating, or lack of eating. It was thought-provoking, and the fact that I had already eaten dinner helped me not feel frustrated because of not being able to enjoy all the great foods being served.

Day 10

More than a week has gone by and I am drifting along into vegan much less painfully than I expected. No doubt that I thoroughly miss animal protein, especially eggs, meat and fish, but I also feel that there are enough options for me to make yummy meals at any time of day. Today, at the suggestion of my health coach, I made a great and very simple tofu and coriander paste. Excellent to use on toast, salads, sautéed vegies, and so on. Simply blend tofu, salt, pepper and fresh coriander in the food processor to the consistency of a cream cheese. I personally like it sprinkled with a little olive oil and paprika.

There are more good news today in regards to this vegan experiment. My energy levels are great and after one week of adjusting, and my stomach/intestines are no longer rebelling against the diet changes incurred by the challenges. It is strange to think that in a month and a half this whole year of experiments will be finished. That will be odd. Although it is highly likely that I will be repeating certain regimes as well as doing food experimentations and trying new food challenges for the rest of my life.

Day 11

I just arrived home from my book-club dinner and am seriously feeling the effects of my food limitations as I write this with a slight buzz. Dinner was interesting… another amazing night of highly intelligent complex women, not enough food, and a lot of great wine. Supposedly, the restaurant was warned that there would be one "nutritionally challenged" woman (me) who did not eat animal based foods. When my beautiful dinner was placed in front of me, I immediately felt my head heat up in embarrassment. Staring at me and daring me to bite into it was a beautiful spinach and ricotta ravioli dish with cream sauce. Vegan? I don't think so. Oh well, wine is vegan. In the end, everyone else enjoyed digging into my meal while I explained to the waiter and apologized for my limitations and asked for a salad. All's well that ends well, and once again I end up feeling a bit drunk after two or three glasses of white wine.

Day 21

Three weeks as a vegan and I have had enough of being a herbivore. Funny that after 4 months without eating dairy, I am not missing cheese or yogurt anymore. What I miss the most is eggs. and I can't wait to make myself a yum omelet! On the other hand, I have been eating great vegan food. Last Friday, which was three days ago, I went with my health coach for lunch at a new place recently opened in Lisbon by a fellow health coach from the Institute for Integrative Nutrition, Ohana by Naz. Wonderful middle-eastern inspired food! I just loved eating various vegan dishes and desserts. The thing about vegan that I find most tiring is that, for me personally, vegan dishes often need to be fairly elaborated to taste good. Thankfully, I like spending time cooking and have a pantry and fridge full of tasty ingredients to play with. Another irritating aspect about this challenge, which is also shared by some other self-imposed food limitations I have tried this past year, is that vegan often forces me to make non-healthy food options. Just consider it: alcohol, sugar and chips are all vegan oks. Oh well. In general I do feel good, have been working out regularly, and am energetic and strong.

Day 28

Oh boy, I feel like absolute crap today. Funny to see how good and strong I was seven days ago, and now, exactly one week later, I am feeling physically weak, mentally grey, uninspired, and emotionally fragile. Partially I think it is physical, since I do have a runny nose as well as an irritating scratchy cough. But also, and maybe not completely disconnected, this last week was the bearer of some disturbing news, including bad health of a close friend and the impending lack of sufficient income to meet our family needs in the face of our quickly dwindling savings. Generally, I tend not to worry or even think too much about money. Reflecting on why this is, I am not sure if it is because I am naturally irresponsible, if it is my upbringing (money was a taboo subject when I grew up), or just my inherent optimism. The simple truth is that I intrinsically believe things will work out financially. But not right now. For some reason, Patrick's and my lack of regular income is making me anxious, tight chested, and in a bad mood. I looked in the mirror today and I don't look very good. My husband thinks that the vegan diet is not helping my overall health, and I agree. But it is almost over. And to be honest, although I don't think I would ever choose to be a strict vegan, these last four weeks have not been as difficult as I was expecting.

Day 29

I am feeling much better today, and getting over my flu, body aches, sadness, and so on. Worked out hard again as well, and it was great to feel decently strong. Which brings me to the conclusion that although I still believe that I need animal protein, it wouldn't be fair to blame this diet regime for my down days. On the other hand, I can't wait until it's over. I miss fish, eggs, and good old-fashioned butter immensely at this point. In fact, it makes me smile and drool just to think about how I am going to break my vegan diet with an awesome cheese and mushroom omelet for breakfast the day after tomorrow.

Day 30

Last day! Woohoo! Started off the day enjoying a couple of slices of seed and multigrain dark bread spread with tofu "cream cheese" accompanied by a green tea. Although it tasted great, the thought of the large and greasy cheese omelet that I will eat tomorrow morning did cross my mind while eating. Vegan, I can't believe I did it! I had originally considered taking vitamin B12 supplements and Omega 3 from fish or algae (EPA and DHA), but did not feel the need. Which means that for the last 30 days, I have eaten exclusively plant foods and nutrients. Entirely plant based prime material for longer than the cycle of many of our cells. Wow! Am I glad that it is almost over? Yes!

Conclusion

Oh boy, I am so proud to have gotten through this one. Never in a million years did I think I could do it! I did learn a lot of new recipes (with tofu and seitan) and so did my husband. I also lost some weight, which is surprising considering that I never went hungry except for the few times that I had dinner out and there were no vegan options. As far as metrics go, considering that this morning I weighed in at 55.7 kg and measured 77 cm around the waist, I lost 1 kg and 1 cm waist perimeter in the last month. Did I like this diet? I must admit that no, I did not. I found that I often had to make the unhealthy choice when eating out to stay within plant foods. Also, I missed some favorites, such as eggs and fish, badly. It was interesting to note that cheese and milk products have somehow ceased to become a part of my cravings. I guess that after four consecutive dairy free months, these foods are no longer a conscious option when I am hungry. In the end, vegan was not as difficult as I thought it would be and there were always tasty options to eat when eating at home.

Regarding how I felt physically, I still think my body needs animal protein. Although there were no effects on my training capacity, sleep, intestinal regularity, or overall mood, I felt a bit off kilter and unenergized, especially in the last week of this challenge. Also, it was the first time since I started these food experiments that people commented on how tired I looked. Which often with the Portuguese, means you look old. Of course my less than fresh look could be for many reasons, including that I have lost a significant amount of weight throughout the year and it may be becoming noticeable on my 51-year-old face. Over this past year, I have also stopped dying my hair, so it is now full grey especially at the front. And finally, the last few weeks have not been easy for personal reasons, which means I am likely carrying a bit of pain on my face. Glad I did it? Yes! Will I continue? No! Will it change how I eat? Yes. Similarly to all the other challenges, it will likely have a long-term impact on what the whole family eats, even if it is simply the introduction of foods that were not a part of our household before. Here are the positives and negatives as I see them:

Positives
- Once again, explored with new foods.
- Found a fantastic authentic Chinese supermarket in downtown Lisbon, with great different veggies and spices.
- Reveled in various nut butters, such as cashew, peanut, sesame, and almond.
- Lost 1 kg in 1 month.
- Lost 1 cm waist circumference.
- Regular bowel and intestinal movements.
- Felt ok at the gym and at training (although there were no competitions during this time).
- Could drink beer and wine.
- Vegan was easier to do than I thought.

- Very affordable diet, especially when compared to paleo.

Negatives
- I really do not like having food limitations, and find that these impose choices which are not necessarily the healthiest. This is a recurring theme, and it feels fantastic to think that this month was the last time I will have to live with limitations for a while since the last challenge of the year will be about time restrictions rather than restrictions on what I can eat.
- Parties and social gatherings were extremely difficult.
- I found it too easy to get really drunk too quickly because of food limitations.
- Vegan can lead to junky eating, as there are a lot of vegan unhealthy foods including all sugars, chips, french-fries, ketchup, corn chips and corn based products, processed soy products, etcetera.
- This diet lacks essential nutrients, such as vitamin B12, fish fats and creatine, which I believe are important for my best mind/body self.

My day off
I started the day with the much dreamt about cheese and vegetable omelet, which tasted absolutely amazing! And for dinner, I made fish soft tacos with guacamole that were oh so yum. Happy to be vegan free!

In retrospect
As I finish editing the vegan month and re-live the experience, I realize that I have something emotionally against this diet. In all fairness, and with complete respect for some good friends that enjoy a healthy vegan lifestyle, I don't feel good after a few weeks without eating animal protein. Although my diet is mostly plant-based, I consider dairy, eggs and fish to be an integral part of my regular foods. Also, I seriously crave red meat after an intense

training session or a long day of playing beach ultimate, and I love to follow my instincts.

There is obviously a lot to be improved in our corrupt and destructive intense farming practices, food distribution methods, labeling legislation, and impressive food waste. We throw approximately 40 % of what we produce in the garbage, and this in a planet where many suffer from hunger. But independently of this, we are an omnivorous species and I think we should be eating a wide variety of foods. I do try to buy organic eggs and other animal produce, as well as bring home the whole chicken from the grocery store, rather than just the chicken breasts. I hope that not supporting intense non-organic farming with these types of measures helps in re-adjusting the balance away from mass production towards smaller more sustainable approaches to farming.

I believe in quality foods, and despair at the fact that quality is often directly proportional to price, which results in many people not having the healthy choice. It is highly frustrating to see the huge contrast in price between expensive wholesome and affordable processed foods. And this social injustice is more extreme in the western developed world. Think about it in terms of eating dinner out. What cheap healthy options are there that allow for feeding an entire family the number of calories equivalent to those that are found in a burger and fries, or pizza, for the same or less cost? There is absolutely no doubt that our current food system is detrimental to our health as well as the health of our planet and that a shift towards a more plant based diet would be greatly beneficial.

For a comprehensive analysis comparing the estimated economic and health benefits of diet shifts towards the healthy guidelines, vegetarian or vegan, I highly recommend taking a look at Springmann et al 2016 and the references therein. In summary, it is currently estimated that the food industry is responsible for more than a quarter of all greenhouse gas emissions, with up to 80 % of these being associated with livestock production. Compared with a reference scenario for the year 2050, a transition towards more plant-based diets could reduce global mortality by 6–10 % and food-related greenhouse gas emissions by 29–70 %. This translates into an estimated economic benefit 1–31 trillion US dollars, which is equivalent to 0.4–13 % of global gross domestic product (GDP) in 2050. I strongly believe it is important to be cognizant of the issues associated with our food industry, especially in the developed world where processed fast food is quick to grab and always the cheapest option. As always, knowledge is key, and we can all make a difference on our health as well as the health of our planet by the choices we make.

To end on a lighter note, this reminds me of a PhD colleague of mine at the university in Toronto, who lived as a vegetarian for 51 out of 52 weeks of the year. However, for one week of the year, she enjoyed hunting and eating meat while camping in the great Canadian wilderness. In the end, I am very happy at the fact that I completed this challenge. Once again, the capacity to stick to it resulted in increased self-trust and a sense of accomplishment. I also realized throughout this challenge that I do have a solid and strong will-power, which amazes me considering that I must have stopped smoking thousands of times before I managed to finally succeed three and a half years ago.

References

Springmann M, Godfray HCJ, Rayner M, Scarborough P. 2016. Analysis and valuation of the health and climate change cobenefits of dietary change. Proceedings of the National Academy of Sciences, Vol. 113, pp. 4146

CHAPTER 12 – INTERMITTENT FASTING

Wow, what a strange feeling it is to realize that the twelfth and final challenge is here and that 30 days from now I will be finished one full year of food experiments. For this final month, I will be doing intermittent fasting and am looking forward to it. Especially because rather than having restrictions on what I can eat, this challenge will be about time, meaning that I will only be able to eat for a limited amount of time each day. There are many reasons why I chose to do intermittent fasting as my last experiment. As you have likely heard somewhere on social media or in the press, there is a lot of interest in the health benefits of periodically going without food for some time. This, not surprisingly, is partially due to the fact that it has repeatedly been shown that fasting significantly increases longevity in various animal species, mainly by slowing down metabolism.

For us humans, the positive health effects of diets that impose periodic caloric restriction, including on anti-aging and reducing inflammation, have turned fasting regimes into a business, as exemplified in https://www.fastcompany.com/3068951/the-business-of-fasting. I personally have used periodical fasting for 24 hours as a reset, and fully believe in the power of these actions for the health of my body and brain. If you think about it, various forms of fasting are a part of most of our religions and traditions throughout the ages. Regarding fasting regimes, the one that I will be following is similar to what is practiced by Muslims during the holy month of Ramadan, when eating food, drinking liquids, smoking cigarettes, and engaging in any sexual activity is out of bounds between sunrise to sunset.

For the next month, I will follow a strict daily fasting and feasting regime where I can eat for 8 hours out of every 24 hours. My regime will be somewhat similar to the fasting practiced by Muslims during Ramadan, yet different in terms of day/night restrictions. During the 16 hours without food, which will include nightly sleep hours, I will not be allowed to ingest any calories. To start this regime, I intend to stick to a schedule of being able to eat between 12 and 8 pm, and starve between 8 pm and 12 pm of the following day. However, I will also allow for flexibility in the schedule to be able to adjust for special occasions, such as a night in which there is a dinner party. If I do want to alter the schedule, I will have to extend the fasting time to more than 16 hours or shorten the feasting time. I can always shorten the amount of time I can eat, but shortening the fasting time will not be permitted. Unlike during Ramadan, I will be able to drink water, teas, infusions, and black coffee during the 16 hours of fasting, but cannot ingest any calories.

There are many fasting regimes with various daily or weekly fasting/feasting schedules, such as fasting every other day, one day a week, etcetera. I chose this regime completely intuitively, as it seemed not too difficult to follow while still imposing a good daily fast. But after googling "eat 8 hours fast 16 hours" I realized that this is probably the simplest and most recommended fasting method for a beginner. The absolute pleasure of this challenge is that I will be able to eat anything that I want. The fact that I can only eat for 8 hours will likely make my choices more important to me, so I am curious as to how I will choose what to eat and how much I eat. Also, I wonder if I can "listen to my body" regarding my eating choices. And even if I do eat well, I worry about whether I will be able to keep myself energetic and feeling good through the fasting periods. Sixteen hours without eating is a lot of time to be on an empty stomach and capable of working, training, playing disc, having fun, and so on.

But then this is it, the final challenge! During this month, I am very curious to see how this year has widened my choices of what I eat. I wonder what I will learn. And although I am looking forward to it, I am also slightly worried about hungry grumpy mornings. Add to that the idea of going an entire month without my much-loved late night hot milk (or vegetable milk) with cinnamon, especially after nightly training sessions, and my anxiety level starts to rise. And yet more bad news, I am slightly concerned about the quality of my sleep, as I tend to sleep badly on an empty stomach. Let us see how it goes.

Day 1

It is now almost eleven o'clock in the morning on the first day of fasting, and although I feel like I have lots of energy, I am starving! Last night, after a couple of hours of disc training on the beach, I enjoyed a nice cold after-practice beer, the last for the next month. Then I came home and had a late-night snack before going to bed, which means that right now, I am nowhere near 16 hours without food. I am very curious as to how difficult it is going be to have the last food before disc practice, and then eventually going to bed five or six hours later and on an empty stomach. On top of that, after I wake up in the morning, I am not sure how am I expected to function for so many hours without eating. Longer-term, I wonder how this regime is going to impact my physical strength, which is decent at this point due to regular strength training and plenty of disc.

According to what is currently known, a healthy meal containing protein is beneficial after training, as it promotes muscle synthesis which in turn is important to repair exercise-induced muscle damage as well as for building muscle mass. I am thinking about this and considering what is the best way to adjust my training schedules this month to make sure I avoid injuries or regression in performance. But first, I must get through today, which means at least one more hour before I can eat! Best to get busy, so I will use the time to walk to the village to take care of some banking and then go take a look at what the butcher has to offer for my first meal of the day. Steak for breakfast seems like a good way to enjoy my first red meat meal in over a month, and a perfect choice considering that I am starving and ready for some cave-woman food and feeding!

Forty-five minutes later on the clock and I am now back from the village with a bag full of chicken legs wrapped up in typical Portuguese sausage (farinheira) and bacon to put into the oven for about an hour. Funny that it was the most attractive food at the butcher, even compared to steaks or meat stuffed Portobello mushrooms. Although I was surprised by my choice, I think what turned me off the mushrooms was mostly the cheese on top. My relationship with cheese has changed, especially lower quality cheeses commonly used in restaurants and other prepared food establishments, which are only partially made with dairy and often have potato starch in them. No longer the unconditional love it used to be, or at least a more selective unconditional love.

Day 2

Exactly what I was afraid that would happen did happen, and last night I woke up in the middle of the night very unhappy and very hungry. It took me a long time to go back to sleep, and in the morning I got out of bed heavy headed and frustrated at the realization that I had to wait at least three hours before I could eat. To add insult to injury, my stomach is not great, which could be because of the different animal foods I ate yesterday or perhaps the to the eating/fasting regime itself. A green tea helped ease the pain in my upper abdomen, but this is not going to be easy and I am starting to doubt if I can do it. Odd that after successfully completing almost an entire year of challenges, I still have doubts if I can manage to complete this month.

Day 4

It is again morning and I am again crazy with hunger. Thinking beyond the hunger, I feel like my brain is highly functioning, similarly as to how it was during the ketogenic month. That makes me wonder if having undergone 30 ketogenic days in the not so distant past has helped my body and brain to be quicker to adapt to burning fat for energy. There are many things running through my mind and my mind's mind at this point, from simple and practical things like food to more complex ones like evolution and the nervous system. I hope I don't bore you as I let my brain and fingers go loose and write. More importantly, and considering my feverish and frantic food deprived state, I hope that my writing makes sense.

One thing is for sure, and that is that right now I am not happy. Not only am I grumpy hungry, I also have a lingering and irritating dull pain in my upper abdominal area, which seems to persist after settling in on day one of this starvation regime. I talked about this pain to a friend who regularly lives with this fasting regime and he doesn't recognize this symptom in himself. And although he has never felt fast induced pain, for me it is real. I can localize it to my stomach and upper intestine, and attribute it to their having to adjust to being empty for such long periods of time. Also, for the first time in all these months of doing various dietary regimes, my intestines are seriously suffering, my bowel movements have not been pleasant, and I have had a fair bit of gas. A self-imposed scatological mess, is what it is!

The difficult part is that there are still many hours to go before I can eat. Although I have periodically done 24 hour fasting bouts before and know what it feels like to be seriously hungry and have an empty stomach, there is a big difference between those isolated experiences and the feeling you get after consecutive days of 16 hours with no food. Now, when I think about it, I recall having a seriously upset stomach for a few days following my last 24-hour starvation bout. To help the time go by, I should focus on what I can learn from this experience. From a psychological and physiological perspective, I am interested in the frantic over-aware state that I am in, which is likely induced by my unhappy empty stomach and intestinal tract as well as a constant state of hunger.

Let me take you on a trip into our gut and let us talk about the scoop on poop. If we think about it, our digestive system is like a tube that travels from our heads to our butts. It is a complex tube with many different compartments and physiological environments, which includes the mouth, the esophagus, the stomach, the small intestine, the large intestine, the colon, bowel, rectum… etcetera. In our well-fed western society, this tube is hardly ever completely empty of food or its remnants. In fact, a significant portion of the remnants of food that we can't digest ourselves serve to feed the trillions of micro-organisms that live in our gut. Regarding my unpleasant bowel movements, I am now convinced that my fasting is inducing drastic changes in the highly complex population composed of a plethora of bacteria, viruses, archaea and fungi that live in my gut, which is likely adjusting to the shock treatment imposed by this regime. It makes sense, and partially explains my current discomfort. To put it simply, my gut's microbiota and the pool of DNA and gene synthesis that these micro-organisms regulate, needs time to adapt to the new unfed and mostly empty environment at the end of my tube. The good news is that I believe adaptation is under way, since I finally had a semi-normal dump today after a few days of serious gases, diarrhea, and mucus yuck-ness. Fingers crossed that it is the end of an unhappy intestinal time.

On top of an unsettled belly and frantic brain, intermittent fasting is having other effects on me. For one thing, I think it is influencing my autonomic nervous system, which is the part of the nervous system that we can't control. Somehow, I feel that there must be a physical reason to the heightened awareness and slightly agitated over-awake state of mind that I am in. Bear with me a moment as I go through my off-the-cuff divagations on this and try to make sense of my current over-very hungry mental/physical state. In our autonomic nervous system, there is the "flight and fight" mode (sympathetic) and the "rest and digest" mode (parasympathetic). However, what mode of our nervous system describes the state in which getting food is the one sole priority? In my view, this is almost an intermediate state, where there is a "fight and forage" energetic need as well as a "calm down and preserve" whatever energy stores you currently have. This mode, essential for survival, I will call the "I must get food" mode, and am sure that it has been a part of our existence and the existence of our predecessors since way before we evolved into a species. And to end this entry, that is precisely the mode I am in right now. In truth, I am feeling slightly overwhelmed as the "I must get food" mode completely takes over my body/brain, and so will try to focus on reading up on the effects of fasting on the autonomic nervous system until it is time to eat.

Day 5

On the fifth day of fasting and thankfully today I woke up feeling a little more normal. Perhaps there is hope that I am getting used to the empty feeling in my abdomen. On a more practical level and from an anthropological point of view, it is interesting to see how tough intermittent fasting is to stick to, even after eleven challenges. Especially because, unlike previous ones where the limits were exclusively on what I could eat and not how much to eat, I am often very hungry and cannot eat. On the other hand, for example as was the case last night, I had to force myself to eat when I was not hungry. Even though I did not feel like eating just before 8 pm, knowing that 16 hours of fasting was coming up made eating a must. In the end, it's a good thing that I did force myself to eat something, since right now, and using a phrase commonly uttered in the laboratory by an Australian post-doc from my PhD days, I could eat the crotch out of a rag doll.

On a positive note, it seems like my intestines and their normal rhythms are getting back on track, and I no longer feel the unhappy and protesting intestinal tract and painful stomach of the past days. Probably because I do feel better, even though I am bonkers-hungry, I am much more positive today and curiously looking forward to seeing how this month goes. One thing that I now realize is that I have to schedule my days differently, and avoid making important appointments in the mornings before I am allowed to eat. For example, tonight I have disc practice from 9 to 11 pm. Since my last meal will be before 8 pm, I will be on an empty stomach when I go to sleep tonight. On top of that, I will have to function tomorrow morning for hours without food. A Muslim friend who does Ramadan every year just reached out, and mentioned that he has played entire disc tournaments of up to three matches in a day without a morsel of food or a drop of water. It is amazing the immensity of the power of our brains, where the perception of effort can be just as prejudicial as the actual physical demand.

Speaking of brains, I have accumulated a decently thick stack of science papers on the biological effects of fasting to go through. I am looking forward to digging in, and considering that I have the excuse that I worked hard today, there could be worse and less productive things I could be doing. When I start to think about all this reading and writing, and the possibility of publishing, I worry whether the content of this book will be interesting for you the reader. Too bad I don't know how you are reacting to the written word, or even if anyone will ever read this besides me. Well, those types of thoughts are not worth dwelling into. Since I can't change what is or will be, they are not time well spent. The one thing that I do like is that I will be self-publishing, which means that I can adjust or change things later, depending on your feedback, if there is feedback.

Ok, off to study what is happening in my body.

Day 6

Intermittent fasting imposes some serious changes in the way that I eat as well as in what I eat. So far, I have mostly been eating high protein and fat meals with some fresh greens and fruits. Almost like paleo but also including high quality full fat yogurts and full fat cheese. I have had one stinky cheese meal, but otherwise no major cravings for cheese, and I have also been eating whole grains, mostly oats in yogurt. About the scheduling of my meals, I am still working on it. What I have noticed is that I eat way too much in my first meal at around mid-day and then as a result am not hungry again until late afternoon. This means that at around 4 or 5 pm, when I am hungry again, I eat a second meal and do not feel like eating again when it is time to have my last meal before the 16-hour fasting bout.

Since fasting is not yet completely natural to me, I have to force myself to consciously be aware and adjust my eating. For one thing, I find it difficult to chew slowly and to leisurely enjoy my first meal of the day when I am ravenous after so many hours of fasting. The other lesson to be learnt is the scheduling of meals themselves. For example, last night after lazy Sunday pickup I realized walking home from the beach that I had 15 minutes before the fasting bout. I ended up running into a small Chinese supermarket and buying an avocado and sesame snaps and quickly chowing down an impromptu plain guacamole made of hand squished avocado scooped up by sesame snaps. Not a bad combination, by the way.

Day 7

I just finished my first meal of the day and it is now almost 2 pm. Breakfast for lunch or lunch for breakfast consisted of eggs, veggies and some whole grain bread. Perhaps because of a friend being over to share breakfast/lunch, or perhaps because of the realization yesterday that I wanted to postpone my 8 hours eating time by one hour (from 12-8 pm to 1-9 pm) to adjust feasting time to end just after sunset, I actually enjoyed preparing the meal before sitting down with everyone to eat it. And so it happened easily and organically... I only started eating after 17 hours of fasting and one hour after the time I was allowed to start. Also, I am proud to say that I managed to chew and eat slowly regardless of my hunger. In fact, I somehow managed to have been the last one of the three people at the meal table to have food on my plate.

Funny how little things can feel like such large achievements. Since cheating is out of the question this late in the game, it is important for me to be able to enjoy food for the rest of this challenge, and I am happy to be getting into the swing of things. Today, for the first time since I started this challenge, I will focus on making sure that I have three decent meals during my 8 food-ok hours. Big meal first, small something when I get hungry later on in the afternoon, and then a larger meal at night. That should work better than what I have been doing. Although I have done very little physical activity, in general I feel good. Brain is on. Like in Keto.

Day 8

Starting to feel closer to normal. The toughest part of this challenge are the mornings, where I have to wait 4 or 5 hours after I wake up before I can eat. On a positive note, the fact that food is a no-no frees up a load of time. Also, although I did not mention it before, my menstrual cycle is completely screwed up, having started about 10 days ago, then intermittently coming and going until now. I wonder if this is partially because of the vegan month, where I used a load of soy products, including tofu, fresh soy sprouts and tempeh, for cooking. What is more likely is that these irregularities are normal pre-menopausal symptoms, taking into account my current 51 going on 52 years. Anyway, I thought I would mention it.

Although I feel much better today, this week has not been easy. Even right now, I have a hollow feeling in my gut and my stomach feels unusually heavy while empty at the same time. At around 14 hours of no food, my needy stomach has gotten to the point of pain, but I can function and not think about it if I get busy. Before going off to live my day, there is one more thing that has been frequently on my mind in the last days. This challenge has made me realize that I spend way too much time focused on food or food related issues. The "hungry human" is probably how we have frequently existed and persisted throughout evolution, where hunger was our normal state. Moreover, even nowadays, a large majority of people in the developing world go through their daily lives hungry. Perhaps because of the partially fast induced ketogenic state of my brain as well as the "heightened awareness" that comes from not having anything in my stomach, I am thinking a lot about this. Let me boldly put it out there... here goes... from a social and economic perspective, maybe the western world would have something to gain if we all went through this experience, maybe we should all be going hungry more often.

Day 9

Today, I am amazed at how normal it feels to now go 16 or 17 hours without eating. After one week and a half of fasting, I am finally feeling good. I am getting the sensation of having gotten used to this regime by mainly maintaining a low rhythm of activity in the mornings when I am most hungry and starting to carry out active life things only after my first meal around 1 pm. Tomorrow morning I plan to go to the gym with my daughter Sara to do a Zumba class at 11, and am curious as to how energetic or lethargic I will feel dancing while starving. Yesterday, I noticed that I have to be careful about how much I eat, as I think that I started eating a bit too much during the 8 feasting hours. Especially highly caloric not great-for-me stuff like typical Portuguese cream pastries (pastel de nata), chips, or ice-cream. After a few bad "giving in to cravings" days, yesterday and today things are back to normal and I am eating healthy foods from all food groups and natural sources. Particularly loving eggs with lots of veggies. In a way, this challenge reminds me of the ketogenic and paleo challenges, as I often choose to eat high fat and protein meals that are low in carbs, especially towards the end of the day.

Day 10

Over the last week, I have been enjoying digesting a small part of the huge amount of scientific literature available on the topic of intermittent fasting. One interesting point is that I have yet to find a negative health effect of intermittent fasting. On the other hand, there are so many benefits that it's hard to know where to start. From stimulating stem cell regeneration to inducing increased insulin sensitivity (which is a serious problem in our society and results in type 2 diabetes), the health promoting effects of fasting are widespread and overwhelming. I also found that there are significant similarities and overlaps between the positive outcomes of intermittent fasting, high intensity exercise and ketogenic and/or paleo low carb diets. Although I am not a huge fan of "conspiracy theories", such as those imposed on the food industry convincing us to eat much more and many more times a day than we need, I do like the energetic and mentally aware state that comes from what I call a "keto brain", loosely meaning a brain that is adapted to being powered by fats instead of carbs. For a great video discussing the effects of fasting on brain function, I strongly suggest taking the time to see a TEDx entitled "Why fasting bolsters brain power", by Mark Mattson from Johns Hopkins University (link: www.youtube.com/watch?v=4UkZAwKoCP8).

Day 12

After almost two weeks, I am now moving well through this challenge and surprisingly enjoying it. I feel physically good and strong, sleep surprisingly well, have lots of energy, and as I already mentioned repeatedly, I feel clear-headed and my brain is sharp. Regarding food, I am now eating well in the 8 hours which I am allowed to eat, and likely come close to consuming the approximately 2000 calories that I normally eat on a day. This is suppeorted by my weight, which so far remains exactly the same as it was at the beginning of this challenge. My son, Tomas, who would like to lose some kilograms, has decided to join me on this regime for two weeks, and is going on to his second day today. He seems to be sliding easily into it, partially because he is on Easter holidays and therefore has no schedule and sleeps in quite late. Tomorrow, I do have a challenge within this challenge, as I have to do an oral presentation at the library in Cascais a couple of hours before I can start to eat. I am curious as to how that will go, and whether I will be able to maintain focus, energy and positivity throughout my talk and during the discussion period afterwards.

Day 13

It was not an easy feat being "on" at the presentation that I gave in the Cascais library at 10:30 am this morning. By the time I left home, I had to dig deep within to be in a good mood and have the energy that my audience deserved from me. But in truth, after eating my last meal at 8 pm yesterday and training afterwards, I was grumpy hungry and drained. Although I don't think that the people that were there to listen to me felt it, I found it very tiring and a bit demanding to talk about healthy fats to a full room while being on an empty stomach for more than 14 hours. Which means that today was one of those days that I seriously questioned myself for doing these experiments. I wanted to eat desperately. Period. Once again, I did get through it and am alive and well. One more chalked down to experience. Even though I have now eaten and am not hungry grumpy, I am still not in the best of moods.

Day 18

It is now 9:23 in the morning and I am so hungry that I keep thinking about that Australian post-doc again, and his rag dolls. It has been over 16 hours since I have eaten, and hopefully I can last without suffering too much. At least another three hours until I dig my chops into that yummy yogurt with banana, nuts and peanut butter which has been nicely maturing overnight in the fridge. Sixteen hours gone and three more to go means a total of 19 hours of fasting! Why so long? you may ask. And the answer is that I have to adjust back to a normal feeding time of 1 to 9 pm after a beach ultimate National league day yesterday, where our team played four games. Since I wanted to make sure I could run around starting at 9:30 in the morning, I stopped eating at 5 pm two afternoons ago (a Saturday) so that I could start eating at 9 am yesterday, before the first game. Taking into account that I can only eat for 8 hours, my last meal was at 5 pm yesterday, just after the last game. So, even though 16 hours of fasting have passed and technically I am allowed to eat, I will try to go as long as I can without food to go back to a decent eating schedule.

Intermittent fasting and my decision to alter the hours for the frisbee day ended up posing a couple of interesting challenges. For one, after my last meal at 5 pm on Saturday afternoon two days ago, Patrick, the kids and I went to see the football game at a bar. It was great to hang out with my grownup kids while all three drank a cold draft beer and enjoyed typical Portuguese snacks called "tremoços" (salted lupines). However, my hot herbal tea just did not cut it as far as the enjoyment factor goes. The next day was game day, and excluding some energy breaks especially in the third game that I think were felt by everyone else on the team as well, I felt ok. My tiredness at the end of the day may have nothing to do with the current challenge, and was surely at least partially explained by the hot sunny day as well as the fact that we only had four women, which means I played every other point throughout the day.

There is a lot of interest in fasting and how it influences physical and athletic capacity, and I have included some references that most interested me at the end of this chapter. According to the literature on the effects of Ramadan on athletic performance, and according to a comprehensive publication by Shephard (2012), there are very little, if any, effects of intermittent fasting on explosive capacity (anaerobic power), measured as sprint speed. There are, however, small but significant fasting induced effects on fatigue, shown as a slight yet significant decrease in performance over repetitive runs in comparison to fed controls. These results are further discussed by the authors, who mention the importance of keeping in mind that the tendency towards greater fatigue with event repetition may be attributable to sleep deprivation or a phase shift in the intake of food in Ramadan fasting athletes, rather than to a cumulative nutritional impairment. Regarding muscle contractile force, the intermittent fasting regime imposed by Ramadan appears to have small effects, especially if hydration, training times and resting times are controlled. Therefore, and taken together, the studies indicate that if sleep patterns are not disrupted and training is maintained, there is little change of anaerobic power or capacity over the month of Ramadan.

That brings me to another interesting parameter that is affected by fasting, brain function and perception. I must admit that this regime has chiseled away at my patience. For example, this was obvious to me during the first beach ultimate game yesterday, which was against a tough opponent and my team played horribly. Even though I am usually positive and supporting, I felt like smacking a few of my teammates and had to take deep breaths to control my temper. There is no doubt that this type of negativity can have an influence on athletic performance. In fact, it appears that fasting has effects on perceived exertion, mood profile including fatigue, as well as the amount of perceived energy by the athletes. Ramadan-style fasting also seems to affect psychomotor performance and vigilance, evident as decreased alertness and concentration. Also, it seems that these negative effects are directly associated to the number of hours of fasting, aggravating as the number of fasting hours increase. Regarding my state during games, I felt highly aware of what was going on at all times. But, I have noticed that I have to put more mental effort into focusing while working out in the last two weeks, a feeling that is somewhat reminiscent from that which I felt while doing the ketogenic challenge.

Conversely to what has been shown for anaerobic power and performance, where athletes show no Ramadan-related deterioration, there is significant deterioration of performance with longer bouts of endurance (aerobic) exercise. It remains unclear whether this is due to poorer motivation, depletion of glycogen reserves, or progressive dehydration. Perhaps this data is related to the increasing fatigue that I feel as the day passes, resulting in lethargic lazy evenings. Reminiscent to how I felt on the ketogenic diet, I am tired after sunset and have to force myself to be active. To sum up how I felt yesterday, during a sports day, I must admit that I didn't feel my best on day 17 of intermittent fasting, although I also definitely did not feel my worst. As a player, I was there, solid and focusing on defense. As I mentioned earlier in this entry, due to my decision to eat before the games started in the morning, my last meal yesterday was at 5 pm just after the games, and consisted of a large hamburger and a cold beer. Sadly enough, I was already feeling an uncomfortably empty stomach and a huge desire to eat just a few hours later, a horrible feeling that was exacerbated by watching my kids and husband eating dinner. Well if you can imagine, hungry then and ravenous now... although I still have a couple of hours to go. Got to get busy cleaning drawers or doing something else mundane but useful. I can't concentrate and am getting grumpy, so perhaps I will go for a walk and pick up some necessities.

Now a few hours have gone by and I am back, feeling proud of myself, and just about to ingest my first calories in over 19 hours. But first a few words. I was having a very hard time focusing because of hunger and decided to walk up to the village and pick up some veggies for a soup. When 12 o'clock hit, which is the time I could start eating, I was in the grocery store. Boy I was tempted to buy a pastry or something to quickly shove in my mouth. But no, I hung in there... and even started cooking a veggie soup with fresh fava beans when I got home. More, I sat down and wrote down these few words before getting my overnight yogurt out of the fridge, which I am now about to eat. Going to focus on enjoying it, chewing slowly and not devouring my first meal in close to 20 hours.

Day 20

Dinner last night with the book-club ladies was interesting and indicative of how socially difficult this regime can be. Since our dinners typically start around 9 pm, I opted to eat before going and sat and drank tea as everyone else ate. None of the ladies even flinched, as they are now used to my monthly gustatory insanities. On a good note, it turned out to be easier than I thought, likely due to the fact that there are only 10 days to go until I am done.

Day 22

Last night, while lying in bed, I was thinking about the reasons why I don't like fasting and made a conscious decision to write things down this morning while they were fresh in my mind. Regardless of how good it is for me in the sense that it makes the good bacteria in my gut flourish while getting rid of the unhealthy ones, gets rid of cells and cell parts in my system that have accumulated mutations, reduces inflammation, and protects against neurodegeneration, the truth is that I feel various negative effects, which seem to get worse as time goes by. For one thing, I am eating much more junky food in the 8 hours that I can eat than I normally do. Partially due to hunger desperation and partially because of psychological factors, I find that I tend to look towards floury high calorie stuff much more often and then think "it's ok, you won't be eating for 16 hours, go for it!". It will be interesting to see how much I weigh at the end of this challenge, but right now I would say that I have not lost any weight at all.

Another negative aspect of fasting is the fact that my mornings are highly unproductive. I generally wake up between 7 and 8 am and can only eat my first meal between 12 and 1 pm. Truthfully, I find that after being awake for two or three hours in the morning, I cannot concentrate on my work due to hunger issues. To add to the negative aspects, I don't feel like using this "unproductive" time to exercise because I am too hungry. In the end, I find myself doing mundane things like cleaning up around the house until I can eat something and get to work. Also negative is the fact that once I do eat, I feel a bit too full to be at my best. But at least I can focus. Yet one more significant issue that I don't like about intermittent fasting is that I am not my sunny self. At least in the mornings and late at nights, I find that I am grumpy. Hungry grumpy, or grumpy hungry. My husband has mentioned it too, and I also notice it in my son who is also fasting with me. He is quicker to explode than when in his usual mode, even considering that he is 16 and volatile.

Day 26

Today marks the one year anniversary since I started this craziness, and to be honest, I am starting to get tired of challenges and cannot wait to be able to eat normally again. My son has decided that two weeks was enough for him, mostly because he had trouble focusing in his morning classes on an empty stomach. He did, however, lose 700 g in two weeks. Regarding my weight, I have no idea what it is but would bet that I haven't lost one gram so far. As far as this challenge goes, I am now decidedly not enjoying intermittent fasting. I realize one of the things I most detest about this regime is the constant stress around time. The having to be aware of what time it is right now, when is the time that I can start eating and how long can I eat for, is driving me mad. I have always hated being attached to the clock, to live by strict schedules, to having to look at the time... alas my choice to be a researcher and now to work as a health-coach. Just knowing that there is a time limit on anything seems to make me unproductive and unhappy. But again, there is a huge amount of discipline involved and that is good. My anarchic self needs it.

Concerning what I am eating when I do eat, the quality of foods in what I choose to eat has improved significantly this week. I am making a conscious effort to think about the decisions I make and not hang onto the "well, I'm not going to eat for hours and hours, so anything goes" kind of mentality. Also, last week, I found that I was getting uncomfortable stomach gases and feeling bloated. After a few days with no dairy and very little wheat, all went back to normal. It is interesting that excluding the first adaptation week, there seem to be no effects of this regime on the frequency of my going to the bathroom.

Day 29

Oh my, I am almost done! And not only this challenge, but a full year of challenges. And oh boy, it will end with a bang! A verified smorgasbord! Why, you may ask? Well, tonight we have my friend's kid from Toronto and his friend staying at our place and we are going out for a celebratory seafood dinner accompanied by cold beers in a traditional Portuguese "tasca" style restaurant. This means that I won't start eating until around 3 pm today so that I can enjoy a typically late Portuguese dinner. And then tomorrow we are going to my cousin's wedding, which means another late-night feast that starts at the church around 4 pm. Like today, I will only start eating late into the afternoon tomorrow, so that I don't have to think about it anymore. Once midnight hits, I am done! All done!

Since tomorrow will be crazy busy with the guests staying over as well as the wedding, and Sunday will not be a good day to measure anything after pigging out, I did my metrics today. This morning I weighed in at 55.6 Kg and my waist circumference was 76 cm. Considering the logistics of this coming weekend (today is Friday), this is probably the last time that I will be doing a daily log. The feeling is strange, I almost feel queasy at the thought that it is over, nerves mixed with elation and a sense of pride. I can't believe I did it! More than one year has gone by and I am almost free of food limitations. What will happen next? How will this experience affect my eating choices in the future? What about my weight? And how will I use different types diets at specific times of life and for achieving specific objectives like muscle building, weight loss or a high functioning mind?

Conclusion

After an entire year of doing food challenges, I had no doubt that I could get through this challenge without cheating, no matter how tough it was or how desperate I got. Also, the fact that the limitations this month were about when I ate rather than what I ate, fasting turned out to be the perfect ending to a fantastic 12-month journey of food experiments. After 30 days, I can clearly state that I am not an advocate of this regime as a lifestyle choice. I do, however, think it is a great way to reset your body, to train self-discipline, or to shake up your relationship with food.

Regarding my weight, no significant differences occurred this month (I lost 100 g) and to be honest, I think it is probably the month that I ate the least healthy of out of the entire last year. Partially, this can be explained by my own internal voice, which excused me to eat whatever I wanted during "feast" hours as there was going to be a long time of hunger coming up. On top of that, the excessive hunger I felt after 16 fast hours often resulted in over indulging. Many times, during my first meals of the day, I would be eating and desperately thinking of what I was going to eat after I finished what I had on my plate. Crazy with hunger, literally. And, when it was my last meal before the time to fast, I ate way too much just thinking of the fact that I knew I wouldn't be eating for a long time. For me, this does not seem to be a healthy routine. Another issue with this fasting regime is that it is socially very difficult. This was obvious by the many complaints from my husband regarding the lack of flexibility in eating hours as well as the various dinners and social gatherings that I went to and did not eat or drink.

The difficulty of sticking to a fasting regime is recognized in the scientific literature, where the number of drop-outs is greater than that seen with other caloric restriction diet regimes. Furthermore, the effects of fasting on weight loss, fat content and cardio-protective parameters have been the subject of many scientific studies, as reviewed in Harvie and Howell, 2016. Analysis of the long-term effects of fasting recently published in one of the most prestigious medical journals (JAMA) showed that alternate-day fasting did not produce superior adherence, weight loss, weight maintenance, or cardio-protection in comparison to regimes of daily calorie restriction. These conclusions were further supported by data of shorter term studies accumulated over the last years, which concluded that intermittent fasting and general calorie restriction diets result in comparable reductions in body weight as well as equivalent reductions in body fat. The one exception to this similarity in results was observed when the intermittent fasting regime was also a very low carb (50 g a day) and high fat diet, in which case there was a greater decrease in body fat when fasting. This, of course, does not take away from the many beneficial effects of fasting on inflammation, brain function, immune system, etcetera. It will be interesting to keep up to the scientific literature as knowledge increases regarding the long-term effects of fasting on these parameters

Personally, I have no doubt that periodic bouts of intermittent fasting can be very positive, having effects in cleansing, resetting, and as a shock to the system. In fact, emerging findings strongly suggest that periodic fasting, together with exercise and an intellectually challenging lifestyle, can protect neurons against the dysfunction and degeneration that they would otherwise suffer in acute brain injuries such as stroke and head trauma, as well as against neurodegenerative disorders including Alzheimer's, Parkinson's and Huntington's disease. However, just like all other adaptations that our bodies manage as we challenge them, after some time under the fasting stress I think our bodies get used to it and the beneficial effects are waned. In conclusion, in my opinion, we should try to keep that in mind when doing any diet of food regime. Also, it is important to remember that when it comes to food, variety and wholesomeness is key. Just like there is a need to change physical training approximately every four weeks, it is not a bad idea to also do that with food as well as any other lifestyle health promoting behaviors. In conclusion, I know that I will occasionally fast, as I always have throughout my life. In fact, on the first day after this challenge and after eating way too much at the wedding, I went to the gym and did an extensive work out on an empty stomach. It felt great!

Positives
   - I could eat whatever I felt like eating.
   - 16 fasting hours meant that there was a lot of time to do non-food related things.
   - Realized that I eat too much and too often.
   - Regular bowel and intestinal movements after the first week.
   - Mostly felt ok at the gym and at training, although I avoided exercise in the morning before breaking the fast.
   - Huge lesson in self-discipline.

- Felt very clear headed and with a high functioning brain, especially in the first few weeks.
- Slept great, even though I was very afraid of this because I don't like going to bed hungry.

Negatives
- This was by far the most difficult challenge socially, as there are no options during fasting hours.
- Felt that I was grumpy due to hunger a lot of the time, especially in the mornings.
- Difficulty concentrating in the last few hours before eating time. Cleaned a lot of drawers and other mundane chores around the house this month.
- Ate too much crappy high calorie foods during feasting hours with the excuse that I would make up for it during fasting hours.
- Found it difficult to manage how to eat and when to eat on physical training and sports days.

My first of many days off
I just have to share with you my two amazing last experiences with food as an intermittent fasting person, which were incredible feasts! The first night, Friday night, which was the second last night in the challenge, we went for dinner at a local and well renown Portuguese sea-food place called Eduardinhos. Wonderful way to spend the last night with my friend's kid that has been visiting, enjoying a fantastic dinner of crab, clams, octopus salad, and sea barnacles served up with rustic Portuguese sour dough bread and accompanied by ice-cold beers. Easy and stimulating conversation with Patrick and four great teenagers while feasting on more than enough food to make it easy to only start to eat quite late on the next day, the last day of the challenge. And then the last day, Saturday, where I only started eating after 4 pm so as not to have to think about it anymore. What a way to start... at my cousins wedding!

The wedding ceremony was held in a wonderful hill-top country home with fantastic views of rolling hills and small villages, just one hour north of Lisbon. It was probably the best served wedding I have been to in ages, and the quality of the food was amazing since it was made in-house rather than catered in. Let me just tell you, it's a good thing I weighed myself before... did I eat, and eat, and eat! Food from heaven, really. Appetizers were served outdoors and included sushi, amazing meats, all kinds of finger foods, Portuguese smoked pork leg (presunto), all beautiful and all wonderful and all allowed! Dinner was a very nice fish soup, followed by seafood crepes, pork with baked apple and finalized by a desert that I did not eat. Then, while dancing and talking, I thoroughly enjoyed the three large tables loaded with delicacies and kept well stacked deep into the night. The first, and a favorite, was the cheese table. Stinky awesome cheeses that I love and that go down oh-so-well with wine. The second was a table full of high-end treats like crab, hams and smoked meats. And the third table served up all kinds of beautifully prepared deserts and fresh fruits, including one of my favorite typical Portuguese treats called "fios de ovos", which translates into egg strings and are made with egg yolk and sugar. I had a couple of plates loaded with these sweet yellow strings and with fresh strawberries, pineapple, and kiwi. Heavenly and like the Dutch say, like an angel peeing on your tongue! There was so much food, that I was happy to hear that all the left-overs will be given to an association close by and then distributed to families with financial difficulties.

In retrospect
It was interesting to re-read and edit this challenge. The almost manic feeling of the first few weeks was especially obvious in the frantic writing, which I edited as little as possible. Perhaps because it was the last of the twelve challenges, and I was therefore likely getting tired of food challenges, this challenge left a strong impression on me. Socially, it was very difficult, and the only one of all twelve that I could not eat anything at dinners and

parties. Also, I have no doubt that it was the challenge that had the biggest impact on my family, not only because of strict dinner schedules but also because it was the one that most affected my mood. To add to the fact that was I grumpier than usual, both kids complained that I often lost focus in a conversation and stopped sentences halfway. As far as the long-term effects of this regime on my eating, I still do not wake up and eat immediately the way that I used to, and now tend to only get hungry two or three hours after opening my eyes in the morning. Although I will not consider this mode of eating as a long-term regime, I will use intermittent fasting throughout my life periodically as a body/mind reset. In the end, I am very glad that I chose to end the journey with this experiment, as it was a true test to my will-power and discipline.

References

Michelle HM, Howell A. 2017. Potential Benefits and Harms of Intermittent Energy Restriction and Intermittent Fasting Amongst Obese, Overweight and Normal Weight Subjects—A Narrative Review of Human and Animal Evidence. Behavioral Sciences, Vol. 7, pp. 4

Nair PMK, Khawale PG. 2016. Role of therapeutic fasting in women's health: An overview. Journal of Mid-Life Health. Vol. 7, pp. 61

Raefsky SM, Mattson MP. 2017. Adaptive responses of neuronal mitochondria to bioenergetic challenges: Roles in neuroplasticity and disease resistance. Free Radical Biology and Medicine, Vol. 102, pp. 203

Shephard RJ. 2012. The impact of Ramadan observance upon athletic performance. Nutrients, Vol. 4, pp. 491

Trepanowski JF, Kroeger CM, Barnosky A, Klempel MC, Bhutani S, et al. 2017. Effect of Alternate-Day Fasting on Weight Loss, Weight Maintenance, and Cardioprotection Among Metabolically Healthy Obese Adults - A Randomized Clinical Trial. JAMA Internal Medicine, Published online, doi:10.1001/jamainternmed.2017.0936

AFTERTHOUGHTS

If you have gotten this far, stop and take a slow deep breath. I just did and it went in and came out bumpy, shaky, and loaded with emotion. As we get closer to the end, I am ever more aware that editing and writing are also part of this process. And although finalizing this project is making me marginally insane and obsessive at times, I also enjoyed remembering each challenge and seeing the whole journey evolve as the days, weeks, and months went by. For the sake of clarity, this whole portion of the book was written over a one-and-a-half-month period after the last challenge was finished, and will therefore have entries from various days. Before I continue my prolific writing mode, I wish I could see what is going on in your mind's eye or your eye's mind. But I can't. I would also love to hear about how what you have read so far has influenced your own approach to food. Has the thought of trying a food regime crossed you mind? What about trying something new when you are out food shopping or going to a specialty restaurant? If not at all, that's ok, hopefully eventually. Regardless of your own food journeys, it is great that you are still here at the final section, where I intend to sum up the entire experience from various perspectives, each with their own sub-titles for structural organization. Enjoy.

Overall health

As you can imagine, there were many times throughout the year where the self-imposed food limitations resulted in awkward moments with friends and family. For one thing, there was often obvious concern for my health, with people that care about me being awry of the potential long-term effects of some of the food challenges. This means that I was often questioned about whether it was a good idea to use myself as a lab rat, or to experiment with something that in the end may have long-term detrimental effects on my health. In fact, there were times that I didn't feel so great, but I consider those to be a normal part of our day to day highs and lows. I tend to avoid going to the doctor, but if I had to self-diagnose the state of my general health through all the food challenges, I would say that I have been in excellent health this past year.

Now looking back, I think I was fortunate to have chosen to do thirty days for each challenge, as it provided enough time for the body to adapt and feel the differences imposed by each eating regime. Also, the thirty day period for each challenge was not too long, and therefore turned out to be a great lesson in my capacity for physical resilience. Except for the ketogenic diet, which had a longer adaptation period, it was impressive how quickly my body rhythms adjusted, regardless of how drastic the changes were from one challenge to the next. Either immediately or at most after a few days of adaptation, my basic body functions seemed to work fine month after month. Regular intestines, nights of undisturbed deep sleep, and mostly a regular menstrual cycle as usual. I did feel that my energy levels varied with what I ate and that this affected my capacity to meet heavy physical demands like weight training or endurance exercises. However, I am merely a recreational athlete and therefore have the luxury of opting to listen to my body and take it easy when I didn't feel that pushing it would be beneficial.

Often, the question arises whether there were favorite challenges, or diets in which I felt better or worse. The answer is that yes, there were positive surprises which I will talk about later. But regarding my self-evaluation of overall health, I personally found the vegetarian challenges to be most difficult on my body. Although I live mostly on a plant based diet, I feel the need for animal protein. The other diet that was physically demanding, especially for the first couple of weeks, was the ketogenic diet. There is a reason for the term "keto-flu", used to describe the tiredness and muscle pain associated with adaptation to ketosis. That brings me to a very interesting point that repeatedly came up when I was doing the ketogenic diet, almost everyone, including health professionals, warned me of the damage that it would do to my health and to my cholesterol levels. This motivated me to do the blood analysis after the ketogenic month as well as at the end of the challenges, with the results shown in the Table below (Table 1).

Table 1. Blood cholesterol and triglyceride levels in mg/dL

	Cholesterol (<190)	Triglycerides (<180)	LDL (<130)	HDL (>40)
May 5, 2015	254	94	150	85
Dec 2, 2016**	290	120	174	92
May 9, 2017	259	89	156	85

** blood was collected one hour after eating a bowl of full fat Greek yogurt with walnuts on day 29 of the ketogenic challenge

The total cholesterol in our blood is the result of the sum of low density lipoprotein (LDL), high density lipoprotein (HDL) and 1/5 of the blood triglycerides (total cholesterol = LDL + HDL + (triglycerides/5)). Although controversial, the measures of blood cholesterol are often utilized as an indication of risk for cardiac disease, with the current guidelines of acceptable levels for each lipid type shown in brackets in the top row of Table 1.

Many consider that the levels of cholesterol and triglycerides in our blood are directly proportional to the amount of fat in our diets. However, according to the scientific literature, this is just not true. In fact, the guidelines for daily cholesterol consumption as well as what is considered a healthy cholesterol level in our blood are currently under revision. What we do know is that all of the cells in our body can synthetize cholesterol and that cholesterol is an essential structural component of our cells membranes. Furthermore, our blood cholesterol levels are more indicative of the cholesterol made by our livers (often from sugars as prime materials) than of cholesterol eaten. Triglycerides, on the other hand, are directly deposited into our blood from the final product of fat digestion, which means that blood triglyceride levels can be directly influenced by what and when we eat. Thus, the reason why blood collection for analysis of blood cholesterol levels normally being done after a period of overnight fasting.

As you can see by my blood work, my cholesterol levels are slightly high, mostly due to very high levels of the good cholesterol HDL. Unfortunately, I hadn't planned on these food challenges going as far as they did, and don't have analysis from just prior to the first month. I do, however, have them from one year before (May 2015) and the results are generally consistent, as you can see from the final analysis done in May 2017, after all the challenges were completed. I would just like to emphasize here that the main reason that I decided to do the blood work and to show these results is to establish that eating 75% fat for a month during the ketogenic challenge did not alter my cholesterol levels! It is a pity that the initial analysis from December 2nd at the end of the ketogenic month were done at the pharmacy with the quick "pricked-finger and blood drop" method. As described in detail at the end of the ketogenic chapter, the results of this practical test turned out to be completely inconsistent. However, after a late realization of the impossibility of the results and encouragement from Patrick to repeat the test, blood collection for proper analysis was done approximately one hour after breakfast. This explains the triglyceride levels being higher than they would have been if the blood had been collected after an overnight fast. On the other hand, and to conclude this part, I was happy to see my latest measures of blood cholesterol, which were equivalent to their usual.

Food challenges and body metrics

As I mentioned at the beginning of the book, I did not choose to undergo food challenges with the intent to change my body shape or weight. On the other hand, although I was ok with the body I did have, I was also aware that I had gained a few kilograms in the last few years, which I partially attributed to age and the fact that I quit smoking three and a half years ago. Regardless, whether it was timing, the fact that I took a nutrition course, the amount of exercise I did and do, or a combination of any of these, my body did change over the year. This was most obvious to me when I took out my summer clothes a couple of weeks ago and things that I love and have hesitated to discard, even though I haven't been able to fit into for years, now fit perfectly. I have charted my body weight in kilograms and waist circumference in cm at the end of each month, and the results are illustrated in Figure 1 below.

The one thing that I want to make very clear is that although I was happy to shed a few kilograms, there was never a point throughout the year that I avoided eating something with the purpose of losing weight. The only time that I did not eat when hungry was when it was impossible to do so because of the challenge at hand. However, I did feel the difference in my body month after month. There was a noticeable change as the extra fat shed off and I got leaner and fitter. The challenge that incurred the biggest weight loss was the ketogenic month, but as discussed in the appropriate chapter, likely due to water loss. This is further supported by the immediate weight gain in the gluten and dairy free month afterwards. Also interesting, is the comparable amount of weight lost in the paleo and vegan months, basically two polar opposite diets. In the end, I lost 4.7 kg over the year and 9 cm in waist circumference.

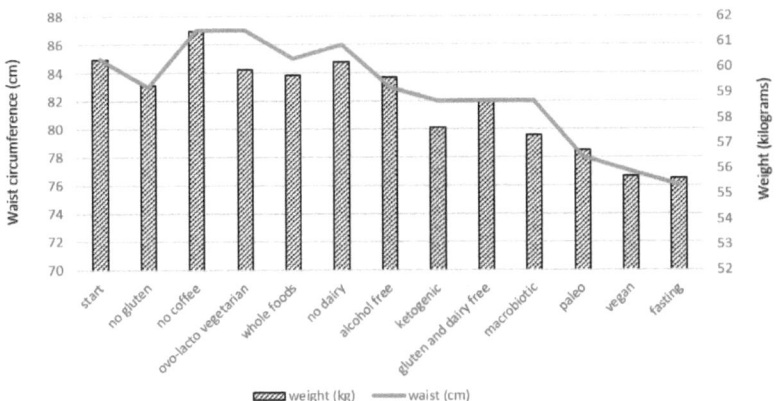

Figure 1. Body weight in kilograms (kg) and waist circumference in centimeters (cm) measured on the last day of each challenge. Over the twelve months, there was a 9 cm decrease in waist circumference (from 85 to 76 cm), and a drop of 4.7 kg (from 60.3 to 55.6 kg).

Looking at the graph of weight and waist circumference intrigues me. I am obliged to say that I believe that the relative weight loss between diets was very much influenced by the time of the year that the challenge fell on. For example, August and December are summer holiday and Christmas months, respectively. This means that during the whole foods (August) and gluten and dairy free months (December), there were frequently festivities and breaks in routines. Regardless of the specifics of each month, I believe that it was the staying power of sticking to the project that resulted in the narrowing down of my waist and building muscle.

Unfortunately, I have dedicated very little time to moving my body in the last days as I work on this book. I find that I eat less, but am also missing the physical strength that comes from putting time into pushing my body. Sitting while I write and edit, I feel my body softening. But that is ok, there are phases in life where balance is impossible for the priority at hand to be met. As I mentioned at the beginning of the book, it was not weight loss that incentivized me to do this, but I am very happy about the results. I feel better and know that I still can be and will be even better. Physically and mentally.

Back to the results as part of the process, I have no doubt that the positive outcome obtained with the body metrics can be mostly attributed to the discipline of staying with the twelve challenges. As far as exercise goes, even though I have always had periods of higher intensity physical activity, I am in general active and have been throughout the year. From the paleolithic month forward, I started incorporation the off-season training from the Ultimate Athlete Project into my weekly routine, and that may have influenced the waist circumference.

Regarding the weight loss results, I think that the challenges made more aware of what I was eating. Also, as a species, we tend to eat a lot when food is available, and the limits forced me to eat less. One more thing that may be interesting for anyone wanting to do consecutive challenges as a weight loss method, is that the body gets used to eating less without "eating less" being the direct imposition with this type of approach. From the standpoint of someone that does not like to be told what to do, like me, this is a good thing. Also, taken together with the increased variety imposed by different limits, the gradual loss in weight may be more sustainable. Once again, I wonder how my journey with food will evolve and what I will have to say a couple of months from now, a year from now, or a decade from now. What I notice is that I eat less now than I used to. Partially, I believe that the higher fat diet that I currently eat, with a lot of nuts and seeds, keeps me feeling fuller for longer periods of time.

As a final curiosity, I did a weigh-in three weeks after the last challenge was completed, and there were no significant differences in my weight or waist in comparison to the last day of the final challenge. I weighed in at 55.8 kg and my waist was 75 cm in circumference, compared to 55.7 kg and 76 cm at the end of the fasting month, respectively. Just as I finish off the book a month and a half after the final challenge, I decided to collect one final weight/waist metrics today. Again, there have been no significant weight or waist circumference changes, with a slight loss in weight likely due to doing less exercise. Now it is time to let go of metrics and to continue to explore with new foods and work the body. Tonight's dinner should be interesting, a vegan wholegrain salad with fresh parsley, celery and blueberries accompanied by a cashew cream sauce. The creamy sauce is very simple to do, just soak unsalted cashews in salted water overnight and then blend with some of the water to the consistency you like. I will add some olive oil, garlic and pepper to the blend to make it tasty for the salad.

The food challenges and (my) physical performance

This is about the fourth time I start to write this section, after reading and re-reading previous renditions and seriously considering removing it all together. I'm not sure of the reason for my uncertainty. It could be because of the relative relevance of this section to me personally, or perhaps simply due to the million things that apply to food and sports dancing around in my mind and becoming so intertwined that I lose the thread. But I must write this, as the biology of sports science is important and something that is very much a part of my life, especially from the perspective of training and nutrition. On one hand, I coach many clients who incorporate intensive physical activity as part of their weekly routines and who regularly have fitness objectives in their lives. And then, to add to that, our physical/mental body and its full healthy capacity is my passion right now, occupying most of my mental space and daily working time.

There is one thing that I must clarify before continuing this section, and that is that I am by no means an expert in sports performance. On the other hand, I am lucky to have three close friends, Pedro Vargas who is just finishing his PhD in sports physiology and who is coach of the national Portuguese ultimate team, Rui Pires, an expert in strength training and human joint mechanics and Tim Morrill, a functional performance specialist and strength and conditioning coach. Not only are these three gurus generally available to me for endless discussions and inspiration, they are also role models for what it means to be an elite athlete, which is not necessarily a professional athlete. Through them, as well as my passion for beach ultimate, I am constantly and consistently amazed about what the human body can do.

Although I am not an elite athlete, I personally feel the need to push my body physically, and train regularly at the gym and playing beach ultimate. Regarding my own training, I am currently following a strength and conditioning routine from the Ultimate Athletes Project (UAP) online platform. This is a fantastic online platform for ultimate players, where Melissa Witmer and her team provide comprehensive off-season, pre-season and in season training schedules and workouts. Also, UAP is always expanding and improving to provide new resources for coaches and athletes. I can proudly say that not only do I do the UAP workouts, I am also onboard as a consultant on nutrition. Which brings me back to food, and more specifically food and athletic performance.

Before I talk about the challenges and physical capacity, it is important to clarify that physical performance is dependent on multi-factorial processes. There is no doubt that food is important, but so is sleep, emotional and intellectual stability, and of course training. The awareness of the importance of integration is key, as is knowing that it is what you do as part of the routine that makes a difference. Back to food and now thinking of food as the prime material, let us consider a scenario in terms of home construction. Everyone knows that a good solid house can be built with less than perfect material. Conversely, a precarious unstable house can easily be built with the best prime material. So yes, eating wholesome good foods as the prime material is important, but it is nowhere near enough.

Regarding the food experiments this last year, I learnt a lot about food and became highly involved in how certain food choices influenced how I felt physically. I also read a lot, and you can find details about how I felt during each challenge as well as what the scientific literature says about their effects on athletic capacity in each specific chapter. Looking over the entire year, my body changed towards a more athletic physical conditioned body. And this, I mostly owe to the discipline of training regularly and eating whole foods rather than to one specific diet. There is also no doubt that I am right now more comfortable with a much wider circle of food choices, and that my eating has changed. For example, regardless of my current objectives, I generally eat more fat and more protein, and much less carbs. I almost don't eat white bread, pasta or white rice, as these are no longer staple foods for me. I am also very aware that I have a tendency for sugar addiction, and now consider sugar a recreational drug and use it as such. That means it is not that bad for those times that I am demanding a lot of my body or brain, like for example simple carbs before a beach ultimate game or a healthy-sugary snack while editing this book.

Regardless of the specific challenges, and common to all, is the relevance and health benefits of eating a variety of plants, including husks (such as cinnamon and psyllium), seeds and spices. Truth be told, plants generally contain chemicals which are slightly poisonous to us. However, small doses of poison from a variety of edible plants also provide amazing health benefits, such as anti-inflammatory and immune stimulating properties. For anyone, and especially for athletes who are constantly pushing their bodies beyond limits, plants and spices are a must. Try making water infusions with ginger, lemon, cinnamon, aniseed, turmeric, mixed as you like or alone. These tasty drinks are great with a little honey, hot or cold, on ice, or to take in your water bottle when training. Other great ways to use spices is to sprinkle them on simple popcorn or baked sweet potato chips. For this, spicy cayenne with a little cumin is a favorite.

As my knowledge on health expands, I become ever more convinced that although there are individual truths and/or periodic truths, there are no absolute truths. And with this, I am not denying that there are alterations in diet that potentiate specific goals, such as for example, protein after training being important for muscle repair and synthesis.

But in the end, the practical aspects of nutrition for performance means different things for different people, with specific goals beng essential to plan eating strategies. That said, everyone, including athletes, should eat good wholesome foods. Foods that are a diverse mix of things that can be found in nature, and preferably as close to the form they exist in nature as possible. Just adjust and listen to your body. Sounds simple, right? In fact this is the toughest part, since nothing is static and we tend to prefer quick results. I heard something the other day that stuck. Digested, it said: no one wants a vitamin pill, people want painkillers. Unfortunately, in my opinion, painkillers do not resolve anything. Not long-term, anyway.

Exploring your body and pushing limits for maximal performance is also about sustainability. Pushing to the limits also needs time for repair. Again, listening to your body is key. Give yourself time for self-care and to heal, to reflect, to fail... take the time to cook and explore foods. In the end, it is all connected. Just to sum up this part, there is a huge amount to gain from trying these different diets for sufficiently long period of time to see how your body reacts and enacts. For anyone, and especially an athlete who is constantly pushing their body to go beyond, self-knowledge and familiarity with foods is a fantastic tool. And this not only from the perspective of feeding the body what it needs, but also because introducing variety in foods increases and therefore optimizes possible individual choices. Positive actions often encourage other positive actions, especially when it comes to us taking care of our physical vehicle.

Balance, limits, and sustainability

I hope I don't come across as high-headed in what I'm about to write, but sustainability is something that I think about often and that I feel deserves mention. Please keep a curious and forgiving mind while you read and hopefully take some positive measures that can make a difference. Also, just to be clear, what is written here is my perspective of things, my opinion, and by no means meant to be an absolute truth. The whole premise of this section is that we, as a species, could work much better alone and together to make this world a healthier and more balanced place to live. Our planet is ageing, and I mean us, we are ageing to live well into decades after retirement. At this point, the world can't afford the luxury of supporting so many old people that are inactive and in increasing need of care for many years. The good news is that there is no doubt that humans can be active and useful to society at any age, and often almost up to until the day they die. Unfortunately, and for many complex reasons, our society does not empower the elderly.

Regarding our planet, the positive news is that each of us can make a difference by making healthier decisions on how we live our day to day lives. This is important on many levels, both personal and societal, as it can greatly reduce the period of morbidity (time that we are dependent on others for care) at the end of our lives. Collectively, we can make an impressive difference by individually taking small steps. And I am not talking about feeding the existing multi-billion dollar industries such as the cosmetic, and anti-aging businesses. Also, I am not referring to spending more time and/or money to find out what could possibly be wrong with each of us as individuals by doing various fancy biotech tests. What I am talking about is the serious need for much simpler individual immediate actions, involving the incorporation of more grass-roots lifestyles. And I hate to be cliché, but more integration. We all know what we could do to better our health as well as what small steps we could take towards environmental awareness and to save our planet.

We are a mortal species, which means aging and death are a normal part of our process. As a quick aside, I must mention a book that I think everyone can benefit from reading by the surgeon Atul Gawande entitled "Being Mortal", where the author confronts the realities of aging and dying in our modern society. For me, aging gracefully and sustainably simply means continuing to learn and to push beyond current personal limits. And this means resisting our natural tendency avoid new experiences and to look towards routines and as we age. This unfortunate tendency for the safe comfortable old shoe has many limiting effects on us, including that we do not expose ourselves to the possibility of learning new things and therefore forget the pleasure of learning. And then, eventually, we start to be afraid of new experiences. Thus, the natural age-related narrowing of our limits, such as physical capacity for example, narrow even more.

I have no doubt of the huge societal impact that would result from all of us actively avoiding letting life take over to narrow our capabilities as we age. Pushing ourselves and consistency is the way to contradict the decay, to lengthen capacity. And since our food, brain, body, and emotional selves are in truth one, we must not lose sight of the "whole person" and maintain a balanced positively challenging life. Eat well, move, sleep seven to eight hours a day, love, laugh, and think about our planet… walk when you can, buy locally grown organic foods, avoid processed, recycle. Of course, not every day is a good day, but in the end, it is what we do as part of our routines that makes a difference.

Are you wondering how this all ties in to the food challenges? Here goes my perhaps loopy logic. Trying different healthy diets is a fantastic example of a positive way to fight the resistance for change. Not only that, trying different ways of eating is a great reason to learn new recipes and to experiment with new healthy foods. Variety in what we eat is great for us and for the microorganisms that live in our gut. And, in the end and perhaps more importantly, the capacity to change and to stick to a plan is hugely empowering, and a fantastic exercise in discipline. Altogether, what I am trying to say is that one small step often results in a ripple effect of good health-promoting behaviors in other areas of our lives. I believe that similarly to it being the small changes in our actions that make a difference in our lives and our health, it is what we do as individuals that makes the difference in society. And it is always worth it and never too late to start.

The diets I did not do

One of the things that became clear to me, especially while editing this book, is how many interesting diets are out there that I did not try. For example, raw foods. If I was stuck on an island with no fire, I would try raw foods, although I don't like raw meats or fish, which means that going raw is just too radical for me. But maybe one day. I'm sure my microbiome would go for a nice ride. Another one is the alkaline diet, which I read up on and didn't think was much different from my regular way of eating. Also, there is something about the alkaline diet that irks me, as scientifically, the levels of acidity in our intestinal tract is quite variable from the stomach to the small intestine, and these don't seem to directly influence the acidity levels in our blood. Thinking further on this, our stomachs' acidity level is equivalent to that of a very strong acid, which could basically disintegrate soft tissue. That said, the alkaline diet advocates whole healthy foods, and I don't eat many processed foods.

Another interesting diet is the blue-zone diet, which is mostly a plant-based diet, and along with some lifestyle characteristics, such as a sense of family, avoidance of smoking, moderate and daily physical activity, and social engagement, is purported to support a long healthy life. Although I did not do the blue-zone diet, is also not much different to my regular diet. Yet another eating style that I did not do throughout this year is the ayurvedic diet. Originally from India and based on an ancient system of life (ayur) knowledge (veda), this eating style can loosely be defined as a holistic approach to health which tailors' foods and eating to three body types for maximum happiness and balance.

I love the idea of studying different ways of eating and learning about food science. Many diets, including the majority of the 12 challenges I did do, have a similar message, which is to eat whole foods. Whenever you feel like you need to reset, try something different for a couple of weeks. A great anti-inflammatory diet is to eat the lowest carbs possible and lots of different healthy fats for a few weeks. Make sure to incorporate plenty of above ground plants and some nuts (pistachios and cashews have too many carbs), but very little carbs and no sugar. In the end, and as I mentioned probably a million times before, it is the process and what you do on a regular basis that counts. And I don't mean that you shouldn't have a goal or a final objective, of course you should. But, in the end, the result comes, whether you like it or not.

Getting back to food challenges, there is something highly enriching about these types of experiments, whether done alone on in sequence. They reinforce the fact that we have the control to define our diet, to choose what we eat. And eating is the most intimate thing we do… to us and for us. Exploring diets and trying new health-promoting foods is wonderful. I know I will try new diets in the future, but for now I need to float free and see where my food-self roams without any limits. Writing and editing this book over the last weeks has definitely gotten me nailed to the sofa. I often look around my ramshackle and funky abode and think about how privileged I am to work at a desk with views of the Atlantic Ocean all around me. I am also lucky that I love to cook and to explore with foods, and therefore frequently go into the kitchen to chill and make food for me and my family. I am curious to see how my food journey evolves and where I will be one year from now. If meanwhile, I don't go crazy finalizing this book.

What Patrick and the kids think

Living with someone with food challenges is not always easy and my husband and kids had to put up with me and my food choices for the entire year. In their own way, they were each amazing at cheering me on, giving support, and bearing with my endless project. Personally, the best part of this was their genuine interest in the experiments and how I was doing, they were my team throughout. I tried not to impose my limits on them as much as possible, but considering that we have at least one daily meal together as a family, typically dinner, and that I cook a lot, in the end our food shopping, cooking, and eating was often at the mercy of my challenges. Their feedback was constant, sometimes good and sometimes not so good.

Regarding the kids, as their mom, I would say that the most difficult thing for them was not having choices they were accustomed to because the choices themselves were always changing. Sometimes that just pissed them off. And, depending on my state, didn't make me happy either. But worth the price of opening their horizons and expanding their comfort zone with foods. They both talk about funny situations throughout the challenges and appreciate the introduction of new, and much loved, ingredients of meals. It was also great fun having them join me in the challenges occasionally, as was the case for Sara in the ovo-lacto vegetarian and the vegan months and Tomas in the intermittent fasting month. In the end, the most important thing for me is that both the kids learnt a lot about good food, real food, and to distinguish that from something that doesn't exist naturally in our biological world.

Patrick was a different story, he was my buddy throughout. He was also often my filter, intellectually and emotionally. And, in those not so few moments that I did not think it was worthwhile to continue, he encouraged me. We also talked a lot of shop, and had seriously rich science conversations. It's difficult to separate out all the parts, it was a whole year and we both work at home, so we share a lot. On a practical level, Patrick was also amazing. He loves to cook and makes amazing dinners. Breakfasts and lunches are not his thing, as he is Dutch and is happy to eat yogurt and bread during the day. But he does enjoy sitting down at the table for my daytime meals instead, and we often have at least one of the kids at home for lunch. Also, everyone in the house loves leftovers, straight-up or re-invented, and we often grocery shopping as a family, so we all live our food together. Anyway, I thought it important to get their feedback on the whole experience and so I asked each of them three questions. Their answers follow.

Question 1- Overall, what did you think about this year?

Patrick:

>I liked it. I thought it was interesting. I enjoyed the fact that at times it forced me to rethink about food based on the culinary challenge of the month and to make meals I would've never have even considered. Long live Google :-) I also liked watching Sofia go through it from a scientific point of view and grow in her knowledge. I enjoyed challenging Sofia at times and learning from the responses. Overall, it was a very positive experience, with perhaps the exception of the last month because the fasting impeded my happy time. More about this in the answer to the next question.

Sara:

>I thought it was challenging not to be able to eat what I felt like at times because it was not in the house. For example, normal bread when mom was going through the gluten free months. But, I did find it a great learning year, and love some of the new recipes and foods we eat now, like zoodles!

Tomas:

>I found it to be interesting. It was cool trying out new foods and learning about the restrictions of specific diets.

Question 2-Which challenge did you like the most and which one did you like the least? Why?

Patrick:

>I liked all the challenges in which it wasn't easy for me to come up with a dinner meal from my usual repertoire. For these, I enjoyed going to Google and looking at what type of things I could make that I would've never thought of and that would fit Sofia's current challenge. I loved cooking those meals. When it comes to the challenge that I liked the least, there is a clear winner/loser for me. Fasting was by far my

least favorite. Mostly because of the way I work. I get up early, work hard, and like very much what I do. But it is mentally intense, and when I'm ready to call it a day, usually around 7 pm, my happy/downtime is often to go to the kitchen and cook dinner. I love thinking what to make, having no deadlines, just focusing on the process. The fasting challenge impeded on that. Suddenly it was 7 pm and I knew I had to make dinner by a 7:45 because at 8 o'clock Sofia could not eat any more. That made my downtime stressful and made it my least favorite challenge, by far.

Sara:

The challenge I liked the best was paleo because I liked the foods around the house like nuts, avocados, and sweet potato cookies. The one that I liked least was ovo-lacto-vegetarian. Since I was on summer holidays during that experiment, I really noticed that my mom was grumpy and missing eating fish and meat. After that, things got better, maybe she got used to limits after this challenge, or maybe I just wasn't around as much because of classes.

Tomas:

The challenge I liked the most was the fasting because we went back to having no limits on the types of foods in the house and on what to make for dinner. Also, it's my favorite because I tried it myself and liked it. In my opinion, it had good results in my weight loss and was not too difficult to do, except for focusing in my morning classes. The challenge I liked the least was ketogenic because it looked disgusting.

Question 3 - What was the biggest "take home" lesson that you got from living with a nutritionally challenged person for a year?

Patrick:

I now look at food differently. I already cooked very international but this year resulted in me becoming even more open-minded. It is interesting that the challenges, which generally meant a reduction of choices, ended up increasing my culinary vocabulary and adding choices (Zoodles anyone?! :-)). I also noticed a difference in my eating behavior because of the things that Sofia did. I have definitely incorporated more vegetables and water, while reducing bread, sugar and juices. Not necessarily because I wanted to lose weight, although that did happen, but simply knowing some of the science and theories behind foods made me want do it, and I feel good about it.

Sara:

I found that it was impressive to see that whatever the diet of the month was, it was easy to get the right types of foods and cook great meals. In other words, there is a lot of different foods available and it is not difficult to try new diets.

Tomas:

No matter what your food restrictions are, it is possible to eat delicious healthy foods.

<u>Loose brain-farts</u>

Dear reader, I just had to put in this section for your, and my, amusement. When I finished the daily logs for the challenges sometime mid-May, the whole document had approximately 25 000 words of unedited text. Today, the day I publish, the edited and re-edited compete book has increased by over 30 000 words. This means that I have worked a lot in the last month and a half, and have had some serious ups and downs regarding my opinion of the quality of this work and whether it ever deserved to be published. Thankfully, I also had moments of clarity and insight. Some of these good and bad moments, which I have labelled as brain-farts, I share with you here before the final words.

Parede, May 10, 2017

It is now the first week without challenges, and to be honest, the feeling I have is a bit odd, like I finished a huge project and now what? At this point, this document has approximately 25 000 words. I hope to double that in the next month, so it is nowhere near finished. In fact, it is halfway there.

Parede, May 13, 2017

Today, the 13th of May, was the birthday celebration of my cousin and close friend as well as her daughter, who is my god-daughter. This yearly event is the same as the one I went to during the gluten free challenge exactly one year ago, which is mentioned in day 13 of gluten free. How delightful it was tonight to attend a dinner party with great people that are so dear to me, and what a pleasure to eat wonderful food at my aunt and uncles' place without food limitations. I even offered them an orchid to thank them for putting up with me as an impossible to please guest at many celebrations over the last year. Also importantly, at the dinner party I had a chance to talk to the Chief editor of a Portuguese non-fiction publisher, who gave me some great feedback on the publishing process in Portugal. But that is for another time. Now I must complete the first version of the book in English and see how self-publishing goes.

Parede, May 30, 2017

Today, approximately two and a half weeks after the last day of the final challenge, I finished the first revision of all the chapters, adding the "in retrospect" sections and inserting as well as formatting the references. The document is currently at 37 500 words, which is perfect since I still have to write the final section, or the conclusion, which I have decided to call afterthoughts. I have also decided to divide the afterthoughts in sub-sections, such as this loose comment part where I can treat myself to mental and verbal diarrhea.

Parede, May 31, 2017

Today I had a meeting with a Portuguese publishing company that may be interested in publishing my book in early 2018. I was nervous, and talked way too much. It irritates me when I forget my own coaching skills. Anyway, it made me think about the book from a more serious business perspective. I will have some decisions to make about that. Meanwhile I have to finish writing the book, then publish the book and THEN see how it goes.

Parede, June 1, 2017

After being in an altered creative state and working frantically on the book for the last couple of days, I decided to take a day off and not even open the document. That lasted until 2:40 pm, which is right now. The main reason to unplug was that I felt that I was losing perspective and becoming too critical. My last read-through yesterday was not a good one, where I felt that although I am the sole author and editor of the entire thing at this point, there seemed to be way too many voices throughout. Although I found the intro to be somewhat light and fun, there was also plenty of heavy and almost scientific writing throughout. Not sure how much I liked it, but as I said, it is almost impossible for me to be objective. Now, after some walking in the sun, a few good meals, a good night's sleep, and some play time, I realize we all have many voices and that it's ok. Hopefully it won't be too dissonant for you the reader (here is the voice of my positive side again, assuming a reader).

Parede, June 2, 2017

Last night after another monthly book-club meeting with wonderful women, I realized I needed to have something in this book about the all the amazing girls in my life and how important their role was in this journey. My girlfriends and science colleagues at the Institute (Ana, Augusta, Guida, and Wanda), who I love to discuss the science of food and the effects of the diets with. My girlfriends from the book-club (Ana, Inha, Margarida, Mia, Monica, Rita and Silvia) who have put up with me being a pain in the neck for one full year of monthly dinners and whose opinions on this adventure I value greatly. The lady friends and teammates from my beach ultimate world (Carla, Constança, Sophie, Joana… and more), who have encouraged and laughed with me throughout. In truth, my girlfriends (Amy, Filipa), and this includes some very close family members like cousins (Ana, Marta, Mia, Filipa, Ana Rita and Joana). My mom-in-law and dear friend, Jos, and my mom, Madalena, were also key in helping me keep my sanity and sense of humor not only through the challenges but also while writing the book. And all the other ladies that I have not mentioned directly, you know how important you are to me. Thanks for being a part of my life.

Parede, June 5, 2017

After a few days without looking at this work, I am feeling slightly more serene. One thing that I can't seem to emphasize enough is the fear of placing a product in your hands that is not up to par. Looking at how big this is getting, I realize that it is going to be impossible for me to edit it to the extent that it does not have some grammatical errors or an escaped word that results in a sentence making no sense. I apologize for that and thank you, the reader, in advance for letting me know when you come across such bleeps.

Parede, June 11, 2017

Brain dump… haha, I guess we have taken a step up the scatological evolution ladder from the brain fart. On that note, if you don't mind graphic sex scenes, it is worth checking it out the music video for Pillow Talk by Lil Dicky. Anyway, regarding my smelly neuronal state, and considering that I am at the final stages of editing and that my brains' seriously gotta poop, what I really want is to share with you today are random thoughts and experiences on the design of the cover for the book.

Initially, I was dead set on having a completely simple black or brown cover with the title in type writer style font. And so it was, the first version looked somewhat like a lab-book or travel log with a plain brown cover just with the title, the sub-title and my name on it. After posting it on social media and showing friends and family, the feedback I got was lukewarm at best. Some people thought it was ok, but mostly my friends and family found it too plain. Then a good friend, Pedro, pointed out to me that my cover looked identical to a google book that does not have a cover. That is what convinced me to change. And considering that I would love this to be a summer book meant to be taken to the park, the beach or the pool, I chose the great combination of colors from the BULA website at www.beachultimate.org. My daughter, Sara, thinks it looks like the result of a kid that was playing on Paint did it, but I like it. Especially after some tweaks in response to feedback from my coach (again) and from good friends from my frisbee life, Jano, Carla and Djuju.

Parede, June 12, 2017

I just got out of bed and am feeling awake and clear headed after an impressive 24 hours of sleeping over the past two days. Throughout my sleep-marathon, I felt my frayed neurons healing and becoming whole again and hope to finish editing this book today.

So much for publishing today. NOT! I started to look at the logistics of publishing and am now feeling deflated. It seems so confusing and scary. My hopes of publishing this before worlds is in France is looking dim. We leave in four days. I am almost ready… or should I say, the book is almost ready. One or two more days.

Parede, June 13, 2017

Today is going to be the day I finish writing. This is likely the last entry. I decided to publish the book on Create Space and it will be available as a print edition on Amazon. Probably tomorrow… June 14 feels like a good day. A couple of days ago at the beach I was talking to my good friend Jano about the cover of the book, and he said, jokingly, that I could put whatever I wanted on it, even a fish, if I felt like it. He used the word "besugo", which translates into a sea bream. And so it came to be. I love the word "besugo", I love eating fish, and it just felt right to add the fish as a final image onto my over-simplified cover.

Parede, June 28, 2017

The final melt-down. Well, I guess June 14 came and went and the book has still not been published. The truth is that I had a complete melt-down while doing the final edits two weeks ago from today, which resulted in me closing the computer and not looking at the document until yesterday. Explaining the crisis is simple... after working more than 14 hours per day on the book for three days in a row, I got this overwhelming feeling of how horribly self-serving it was. And maybe too personal. I closed the computer and went to bed at 5 am, convinced that I would not publish it at all.

Thank goodness for time and for how it brings things into perspective. After my crisis, I had the huge advantage of going to France for the World Championships of Beach Ultimate in Royan for ten days. The tournament was awesome! Thirty-eight countries not considering the mystical Currier Island, 1700 players, over 200 staff and volunteers, hot sunny sandy days, and amazing beach ultimate. As far as food goes, I thoroughly enjoyed eating loads of wonderful smelly cheeses and fresh seafood, especially oysters and mussels.

Now I am back from France and able to think clearly again. I hope to publish in the next few days before heading to Meco for the 21st rendition of the Bar do Peixe tournament just 40 km south of Lisbon.

Reminiscing about one year back, after arriving in Lisbon from World Clubs in London and going to the 20th rendition of BDP while doing the coffee free 30-day challenge, makes me think how much has changed since. If nothing else, this work is a testament of a wonderful year of food experiments, learning, and thinking. I hope that my voracious reading has helped me to be somewhat capable of transcribing what I have learnt this past year to you, the reader, in a fun and pleasant manner. Thanks to my book-club and especially to a great new friend Margarida (Star) and a great old friend Silvia, some of my recent favorite authors are Paul Auster, Chimamanda Ngozi Adichie and Jonathan Franzen.

It has not been easy to be sole editor, and many may think I am nuts not to give this to someone else to read over. On one hand, I would love someone's opinion. On the other, this way I assume full responsibility. I hope that you can forgive me for escaped grammatical errors, bad editing, or nonsensical phrases, and that they don't interrupt the flow of your reading to the point that it becomes not enjoyable. My number one worry is that I may offend someone by my written word. I hope my opinions and experiences are not taken personally. Also, please realize that if you are a part of my life, you are part of this work, whether you are mentioned or not. Am I proud to be done? Hmm, not sure… I am expectant to see what happens next. But positive, after recuperating from a periodic negative mind-state, overall feeling positive and looking forward to your feedback.

Parede, June 30, 2017

Last entry? Already in Create Space and now building the book. Not too difficult, thanks to their step-by-step process. Anyway, it is now very late on Friday night, and as I construct the actual book the content itself becomes anonymous. It is now a whole different thing. I like to think that this book is part of the base in my personal path of growth. It feels right to do it. My close friend's son said something interesting that now comes to mind. He said, "If you want to make a difference locally, work locally, and if you want to make a difference in the world, work globally". I believe that I can make a difference both in my community and in our world, starting with my family. People have a lot to teach, life has a lot to teach, and everyone has a right to health.

Parede, July 4, 2017

Today is the day. After a soul-filling and body-abusing weekend at Bar do Peixe (BDP) and sleeping on the beach with my favorite dude by my side, the book is ready… and so am I.

FINAL WORDS

Final words, so many words. At this point, and after wrapping up all the specifics and small bits as much as possible, I am going to take the mental and literary space to widen the perspective of this book beyond the food challenges. Bear with me as I put this out there for you. As single writer and editor, I have repeatedly read and re-read, lived and re-lived, edited and re-edited this work. It can be a lonely job, and one that takes me on a mental and emotional roller coaster as I vacillate between elation and apprehension about the quality of the work as well as at the possible outcomes of the next steps. As publication becomes a reality, the Portuguese word "obra" keeps coming into mind. I can't seem to find an appropriate English word as a substitute for "obra", which google translator returns as; work, job, doing, or shell-work. Personally, I can think of a few more options, such as; project, construction, construction site, and construction product.

What attracts me most to the word "obra" is that, in the Portuguese language, it simultaneously translates into both the unfinished construction site as well as the final constructed product. Although I feel good about the completion of this work and trust that it is now ready to put out there, it somehow rests my mind to consider that changes are possible, and therefore that it is a work in process rather than a final static and immortal piece of crap. As I spend hours upon hours and days upon days on this, and try to hold onto my sanity and objectivity, that is the one thing that relaxes me. The possibility of future improvements, as you, the reader, give me feedback. On a more grounded note, and back to the word "obra", this word is typically used to define the product of a creative process such as a book, a painting, a work of music. In the last few days, I have had plenty of time to think about this "obra", and especially about how I would like this final section to develop.

Yesterday was particularly productive, since I had to take care of bureaucratic practical necessities, I was lucky to gain the mental space for a couple of serial brain farts while taking the train, walking, and then waiting for five hours in a government office to renew my ID. Sometime after taking my ticket and waiting in ID renewal place, I realized it was taking close to thirty minutes per person and I had thirty-nine people in front of me. Considering that the government office closed at 5 pm, the math told me that I would not be served that day. As I was ready to leave, an amazingly patient and smiley public worker told me that no-one that sticks around goes home empty handed. My ID had expired and I needed it, so ok, it was going to be a long day. Since I hadn't brought a computer or a phone and my brain was spinning with ideas, I walked down the street to a small store to buy a pen and paper, went back into the government office and found a chair in a quiet corner to sit and work at.

It felt great to write down lists and flowcharts and loose phrases connected by lines, while trying to put sense and order to my thoughts. After a few hours sitting in a corner of the full government office working and periodically exchanging silly comments about the absurdity of public services with my awaiting neighbor, I finished my list and proceeded to have an enriching anthropological day. I would have loved to have a camera filming my tiny corner of a Portuguese public office for five hours. The people made the day. As usual, I am always and eternally amazed by people. We are all so the same and yet all so different. When I left, I felt like hugging everyone and wishing them a great life! Moreover, this section was drafted during that time and ready to be finalized here.

Before I go off on my divagations, I think it is worth going into some overall leftover and all-encompassing feelings and opinions about this year, and to tie some loose ends and sum up the experience. One issue that I think is important to talk about is the topic of cheating, or rather not cheating and sticking to doing what I said I would do during each challenge. Besides the few unintentional slip-ups in the gluten-free month, I did not waver from doing what I said I was going to do for the rest of the year. This, for me, was a huge point of honor. And, to be honest, I was surprised. In the end, the persistence to stick with the project as the days, weeks, and months passed turned out to be immensely empowering for me, and I am now sure the growing sense of self-trust gave me the strength to face new challenges. I also realized that I have way more will-power than I thought, and much more discipline. Or I did for this project, anyway. I have always tended to be decadent, of giving into my desires and doing what I felt like rather than what I know I should do. At 51, this journey was a fantastic lesson in discipline. Even taking into account occasions where I seriously questioned what my intent was, or during those times where I felt what I interpreted to be negative physical effects of certain diets, I stuck with it. I will discuss this more later, and how I think it can apply to life.

The actual order of the consecutive challenges is another point that is interesting and worth discussion. I have often thought about whether things would have been different if the order of the diets had been different. Maybe. I have no doubt that my perception of each of the challenges was very much influenced by the time of year as well as the immediate physical demands on me at the time. For example, macrobiotic in the dead of winter was like a warm hug on a cold day, and paleo in spring and together with increased physical training was a powerful surge. In the end, I am very happy that the order of the challenges was as it was. Furthermore, I also like that each was dictated based on immediate criteria of how I felt at the time, to the point that sometimes the choice of what to do next was decided on the last day of the preceding month. For example, I remember being very edgy during the last week on the ketogenic diet and snapping at my coach when she suggested I try paleo next. As valid as her arguments were, I felt that I needed carbs after keto and therefore chose to follow it with a gluten and dairy free month. I am now sure that the capacity to choose each challenge up until day one of that challenge helped me stay motivated. As time passes, each individual month will likely blur into each other. No, that does not mean I will forget what I learnt, but rather that isolated moments and details of specific moments will fade as personal and practical lessons learnt throughout the year are expanded upon.

Month after month, it was great to share my challenges with my friends and family. Not only were they supportive, they were also very interested in the specifics of the diets that I was doing, how I felt, how much I liked each challenge, what I ate, etcetera. The one question that most people asked was, "which one was your favorite challenge?" To answer this and looking back on the entire year of all twelve food regimes, there were some unexpected surprises as well as lessons that will forever change the way I eat. I believe that the comments in each of the specific chapters show that there were good and bad moments in all the challenges. But overall, I was most surprised at how much I enjoyed the paleolithic diet. Considering that I don't normally eat that much meat, it was amazing how much I liked it. I also did not expect the way my body reacted to a vegetarian diet, and it made me realize that at this point in my life I need some animal protein to feel good. As far as long-term changes or take-home lessons, I now eat much less carbs than I used to. I don't mean that I am eating a lot of meat, as I continue to enjoy mostly a plant based diet. Rather, the changes are mostly that I do not eat much wheat, with my starchy carbs coming mostly from nuts, legumes and whole grains.

The biggest thing that changed in my eating is an obvious increase in the flexibility and variability of foods and eating styles. I notice that I eat differently every day, and the amount of carbs I eat is very much associated with how much physical exercise I do in a single day. For example, I eat an almost ketogenic diet when I spend my days sitting behind the computer, and eat carbs, especially simple carbs like pasta or rice, mostly just before, during or after doing some strenuous exercise. Don't get me wrong, this way of eating is not strict or even regulated, rather it seems to come naturally right now. For example, I have noticed that as I use my brain a lot while writing, I crave sugar. I happily give into my cravings, ensuring it is the good stuff and in moderation. Spicy and fruity infusions are awesome, for instance, with a little natural sweetener like honey. But back to the question of which one was my favorite, the answer is that none was and all were. I am sure that the lessons learnt will lead down different paths as time goes by, and that this wouldn't be possible without the whole trip.

Before I move onto words that will try to concretize my abstract thinking, and on a more serious note, there is something I stated at the beginning of the book and that I feel I must reiterate now. The contents of this book are not meant to be taken as scientific literature, as it is by no means a science document. All the scientific discussions herein are sprinkled with my opinion and experience. And valid as those may be, they are not "truths" but rather a compilation of my thoughts, feelings, and subjective life. Don't get me wrong, I do believe that this can be an important document, and hope to have been capable of pleasantly transmitting some science to you the reader. Better yet, I hope to give you the desire to study further and explore your own personal food self. I strongly suggest to anyone who wants to learn more about the science discussed here, that they take a look into the original literature using an appropriate search engine like NCBI (https://www.ncbi.nlm.nih.gov/pubmed/). Considering that we are now in the summer of 2017, the references provided here are a good place to start. As a health professional, I think I would have enjoyed reading this book, and so hope that other health professionals find it interesting and worth their time. I am, however, very aware of its imperfection, and would rather think of it as a perfectly imperfect or imperfectly perfect piece of work.

Ok, here we go. I believe I saved the best for last. Bear with me if my mental thread gets too convoluted and long as I go from the concrete specifics of the food challenges to the abstract generalities of life. And please also understand that by no means do I claim that what I am to divagate on is based on exclusively original thoughts. This is simply not the case. Rather, my mental thread is the result of much learning based on reading, experiencing, thinking, living, as well as a mish-mash of many others things not mentioned specifically. As an example, I mention various friends and family members and cite many scientific references in the book, but there are many more that I have not included. For those not mentioned, which as I said there are many, please know that I extremely grateful. I hope I succeed in intercalating the concrete aspects of this "obra" and to relate these to the much more random and abstract lives that we live in this strange and singular spinning planet.

The first point I would like to discuss that is not directly related to the practical aspects of this book is the actual process that allowed for its completion and how that process applies to us and our lives. We humans, most of us, or rather all of us, always or at least at times tend to be very much result oriented. It is the perspective of achievement that mostly drives us. This result oriented mode of operation comes with a series of problems. There is no doubt that we need objectives and/or goals, we obviously do, and ideally realistic ones. But that does not take away from the argument that there are serious downfalls to being too focused on the result. To make my point, I would like to take you back to another construction analogy and to consider the pyramid. When on its correct side, which is the base, the pyramid is highly stable. However, turning it upside down causes it to topple. That is what I think happens when we focus on the result (the top of the pyramid), rather than the process (which starts wide at the base and slowly works itself towards the top). In our personal projects, we tend not to enjoy building gradually towards sustainable pyramid-like structures. Unfortunately, and maybe because of my mood right now, I see the inverted pyramid as a huge problem in our existence, personal, societal, political, and financial. Just think of the highly skewed distribution of money or power amongst us. And the few that have a lot, typically want more. Ok, maybe that is too dark, and I am not that person. I am happy and adjusted and want to focus on the process. Let's get back to the process.

I will take the liberty to use the completion of this "obra" as an example. As I am starting to see the possibility of completion, I am at awe at the immensity of what is actually feasible. But only because of the sum of all components, as it was built in parts, in baby steps. Looking over the daily logs, there were good days, mediocre days and bad days. In the end, it was the consistence and persistence that made finishing the project possible. Basically, it boils down to doing a bit every day until it stops, and this particular work went on for long enough to mature into this product. Undoubtedly this is dependent on internal as well as external factors, including perseverance to not give up, patience, forgiveness of failure, and support and encouragement from others. Having a clear vision regarding where we want to go and allowing for adjustment based on objective analysis and feedback is key. As anyone who is knowledgeable in coaching knows, be it collectively or individually, long-term objectives should be broken down into more immediate goals that are reachable. If the focus is solely on the final result, the truth is that once the result is reached, and life goes on, there is not enough ground work done for further construction. Funny that we just love the concept of a quick success, the glorified hero idea. When in truth, the result is never as simple as it seems.

Allow me to get a little repetitive in making my point about final results by reiterating why we need the process and why victory is often anti-climactic. I can clearly see at least three oversimplified scenarios which frequently happen when we focus to much on achieving a final goal, as individuals as well as in society. The first two are assuming success is reached. So the goal is met... and then what? It is day to day that we live, and the satisfaction received by reaching a desired goal, or a win, is at best an intense but relatively short-lived pleasure. By short lived I mean that, by itself and in isolation, the win is not enough to keep us satisfied long-term. So, to put it bluntly, the first negative scenario is the "one-trick-pony" type of success, which normally results in disaster down the line. Conversely, when a goal is reached as part of the process, it is a sustainable result, and empowers us to take another step towards the next, more ambitious, result. And thus, the process continues.

Another and second possible negative effect of being too result oriented is not living fully and with complete clarity but rather being driven by single-minded ambition. As I look around and get critical about society, it saddens me to realize how many of us are obsessed by what we think we want, and then end up living a life that is not at all what we actually wished for. Or what we expected it to be, for that matter. This sad phrase comes to mind: you wanted what you have and now want what you lost. We forget that we change. When we focus on the results sole mindedly, they can end up controlling us, and it should be the other way around. We need to control what we can, imperfectly, but consistently. Moments of doubt, failure, instability, and regression, all are ok. In fact, they help us to reestablish our goals and to lucidly face what we must do, what we have the capacity to do, which changes.

There is yet a third and probably most common negative outcome of focusing on the result alone, and that is failure. And not just failure of achieving the goal, but also failure to continue to fight for it. As I see it, this last option is most common. Most failure comes from giving up when we don't see the results we want, or when things are not moving forward as fast as we would like. Which brings me back to our attraction for the pain-killer as opposed to the vitamin pill, a keystone of marketing strategies and exemplary of our society today. Often, we don't consider that giving up is failure. Nor do we consider re-scheduling the initiation of a project, or finding yet another more exciting and often impossible substitute goal to try to reach, to be failure. But the inverse of failure, success, like most completed "obras", takes time to build. A successful accomplishment is partially due to the establishment of longer-term goals, but mostly to persistently and directionally taking the small steps that allow for slowly moving towards these goals. There are always bad days, progress never occurs in a linear manner…so again, staying conscious of decisions and taking time to repair is important.

I was often asked how I could deal with having specific food limitations for 30 days without rest, wasn't it just too difficult? In truth, it became less difficult as time went by. Each day, week and month was not isolated, but rather built on each other. And that is one very positive aspect of this year. Via the food challenges, I pushed beyond my limits physically, emotionally, as well as intellectually. No doubt that there were tough times, but the learning curve was huge and made the effort worth it. For example, the fact that I could hardly do exercise for the first three weeks of the ketogenic diet, having to deal with food limitations and drinking too much at social situations, being manic and insecure as I compile and finish this book... and these are just a few of the many hurdles that had to be overcome. I try to satisfy myself that even if no one reads this, it was worth the trip for me and my family. I feel that I have gained the strength for many more experiments and challenges and look forward to them.

When I recall the original concept of this book, it is lovely to realize that the initial goal was to do two gluten-free weeks. It was precisely meeting that goal and the positive experience to get there that boosted the desire to expand the challenge to one month, and then to try more challenges. It was only after four or five challenges that the idea of writing a book arose, and only at around month eight to do a full year of challenges. Celebrating each small achievement, adjusting goals based on mindful decisions, taking time to digest acquired knowledge, acceptance of ourselves and our flaws, that is what makes us balanced and happy people with balanced and happy lives. Balance... equilibrium... for us and in our lives. Because time doesn't stand still, these are transitory states. Which brings me to another one of my favorite topics. Our need to push beyond current limits for change and growth to occur. We are all aware of "having gone too far", be it physically, mentally, verbally, emotionally, or in any other sector of our lives. There is a point at which we go beyond what we are comfortable with, we have inevitably overstepped our limits. Sometimes, we can even cause damage and lose some serious ground by going too far beyond. But mostly, this overstepping of our limits is internal and allows us to establish new limits. Expanding our comfort zones and establishing new limits can therefore be positive, and permits us to set new and more challenging goals, which is a needed aspect of sustainably,.

It's amazing how much of our lives are at the mercy of our perception. Our mind and the mind of our mind and our capacity to harness their awesome capabilities is what rules us. How we think, our perception, affects our actions, and what we do affects how we think. And not necessarily in that order. That is why challenging ourselves gives us self-trust and strength to do more. Think of this in terms of travel, and how we feel about being in a completely strange new place. Is it a good or a bad sensation? If approached from a traveler's mind that wants to explore and learn new cultures, it is very positive enriching experience. However, being in a completely foreign place can also bring fear, insecurity, and loneliness. How we perceive change is key. And experiencing change itself, succeeding at managing it and learning from it, gives us the confidence and desire to explore a little further. In the case of this book it started with food and the fact that the challenges were self-imposed. As momentum was gained with the capacity to do one thing and expanding the comfort zone, the desire to go on was spurred. Food but not only. Because like everything else in our lives, one sector trickles into another and so on and so forth.

We humans need to have projects. It is the planning, anticipation, interest, novelty, and fight that keeps us alive. In the end, the food challenges turned out to be a fantastic project, since the one thing that we can control is what we put in our mouths. Just like there are no absolute truths, some of the common "wisdom sayings" out there also irk me. For example, I just saw one today that stated, "You have everything in you to deal with whatever challenges life throws at you". If that is the case, then why are there so many unhappy and unbalanced people? Crumbling with the weight of life, in a society that does not accept or empower aging or death although it is an integral part of life? That is why I do think we, and our planet, can gain a lot by us taking control of what we can control. Another saying, commonly used to empower people, is "You are in control of your life!" Without some clarification, this one also irritates me, as it forgets to consider inevitable and unpredictable life happenings that are completely external to our control. In fact, those are exactly what I use to work on my personal spirituality. Not making decisions based on avoiding pain, and learning to recognize and accept the things that I cannot control, to release these from my active involvement, and to trust in the future.

The final paragraph is here, and I would like to end in my typical optimistic fashion. A couple of days ago at the supermarket, I saw a Portuguese novel by Helena Sacadura Cabral, which the title loosely translated into: I like to like. I stared at the title and for some reason it resonated with me, and made me think that I like to like my life, my family, my friends, what I do. And that this "liking to like" is very different from simply liking those same fundamental parts of my life, which I also avidly do. Thinking further on this, I believe that liking to like is something we can all work on. The truth is that we are largely in control of what we do, and definitely in control of what we eat. As we discussed earlier, our actions are an integral part of the feedback loop that formulates what we think, which in turn empowers what we do, and endlessly feeding back to the process of thinking and doing and doing and thinking. From a concrete and practical perspective, that is why it is the actions that we take in our daily lives that forge our paths. Our actions and their associated mental processes are what give us the confidence in ourselves to go sustainably beyond our current comfort zones and to be happy and balanced. And, as I mentioned before, nothing human is simple. Be it food, physical exercise, learning or teaching a new skill, travel, or any other action that results in enriching change, the effect is to empower us to go further in other areas of life. And that, for our integral minds/bodies as well as for our planet, is always worth it.

ABOUT THE AUTHOR

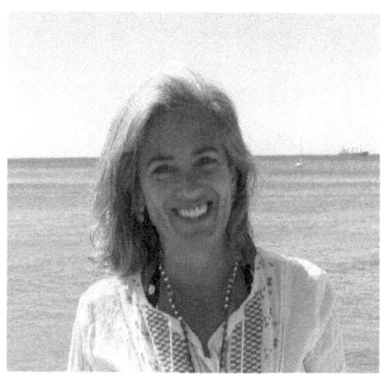

Sofia lives in a small sea-side village just outside Lisbon, the capital of Portugal. She is currently a health coach with clients from all over the world and is involved in research projects at the University of Lisbon. "The Food Anthropologist... a one year journey through food challenges" is Sofia's first book. With a long-term research background, a PhD in biology/genetics (York University, Toronto, Canada) and a health coach certificate (Institute for Integrative Nutrition, New York, USA), Sofia is highly interested in food as the building blocks of our bodies and brains, and the effects of our behavior on our physical and mental health. For more information about the author, check out Sofia's website at www.besthealth.life.